SUCCESS STORIES

Note on Success Stories
The following success stories are voluntary testimonials of people affected by obesity or diabetes who participated in the NaturalSlim program or applied the knowledge acquired through reading the books *The Power of Your Metabolism* and *Problem-Free Diabetes*, or from the videos of Frank Suárez's MetabolismoTV channel on YouTube, with the purpose of learning how to restore their metabolism and slim down. As a note, NaturalSlim, MetabolismoTV, and Frank Suárez do not treat or claim to treat diabetes because diabetes is a serious disease that requires the expert supervision of a physician. What happens is that, by improving the efficiency of metabolism, people lose weight and as an additional result their diabetes is controlled, along with other obesity-related conditions such as high blood pressure, cholesterol, and triglycerides. People with diabetes need to be cleared by their physicians to be accepted into the NaturalSlim program. As a result of their slim down program, these people learned and applied the same techniques for metabolism restoration, plus the "lifestyle" taught in this book. It is worth noting that many of these individuals had the added benefit of the personalized follow-up and support of a NaturalSlim Certified Metabolism Consultant until they achieved their personal goals.

"I am from Costa Rica, and I am 44 years old. Three months ago, I made my debut as a diabetic. I went to the emergency room at the clinic with a glucose level of 628. I was tired, I could not see well. I did not want to exercise, and I ate a lot of carbohydrates like crazy. When I was diagnosed with diabetes, the treatment was two metformin and 10 units of insulin in the morning. I bought the book The Power of Your Metabolism and started listening to Mr. Frank's audios. I started with the 3x1 Diet and the Problem-Free Diabetes book. I have been taken off insulin and metformin. I have lost 44 pounds (20 kilos) and I exercise without any problems. I have more energy. I have gone from a 24-pant size to a size 12. I am very grateful.
-E. Vargas

"I feel great, my clothes fit very well. I have already discarded all my plus-size clothes and bought new ones. I went down four dress sizes and realized that wheat was my aggressor food, thanks to MetabolismoTV."
-S. Liliana

"I entered the program because of my health and overweight since I was a size 40 waist and continued to gain weight. Now I am a size 34 and I no longer need to use medications for diabetes or high blood pressure. People ask me all the time when they notice the change. Since I now have a lot of energy, I am in the gym exercising frequently after improving my body's metabolism. I do not feel like I am on a diet, it is a lifestyle. I have recommended it to many people, and it has worked for them too."

-W. Medina

"Thanks to God and your advice I have managed to lose 43 pounds (20 kilos) and I'm going for more! I want to thank you for what you do to extend one's life. I no longer have high blood pressure, no more high blood sugar, no more depression, no more anxiety. I've had my pills cut in half and I am grateful."

-I. Rodriguez

"Eight months ago, I decided to change my diet: no sugar, no flours, no dairy. I weighed 120 kilos (265 pounds) and I lost 25 kilos (55 pounds) with my dear Frank's diet and of course with a lot of willpower. Yes, you can!"

-Y. Lopez

"In January 2017 I decided to make a change when I noticed that I couldn't tie my shoes to go to work and that the steering wheel of my truck was almost reaching my belly (stomach). I started with short daily walks watching what I ate and understanding that not everything that looks good or tasty was healthy for me. Eventually, I found Mr. Frank Suárez of MetabolismoTV. Today I feel like a new person, I can buy the clothes I like, and I keep learning day by day. I lost 70 pounds (32 kilos) in five months. My life before was to come home and sit on the couch to eat, today I come home and change to go running or to the gym. Cheer up, victory is just a step away."

-M. Gonzalez

"I wore a huge size 18 in clothes and a size 3x in blouses. I had high blood pressure and diabetes, which was the main reason for seeking help. My diabetes and high blood pressure stabilized so much that today I do not have to be on medication. As of this date I am a size 10 and wear size medium blouses. I feel happy."

-Z. Vallejo

"Your book saved me from a cruel fate! When I started this change, I was 40 years old, 5' 7" (173 cm) tall, and weighed 220 pounds (100 kilos) with an abdominal circumference of 49 inches (125 cm.). I was a size 48, with high triglycerides and high blood pressure. I would get tired, and my hands would fall asleep. Today, I weigh 161 pounds (73 kilos), with an abdominal circumference of 32 inches (81 cm.), I am a size 32 pants. I have a lot of energy, my hands do not fall asleep, and I feel great. One of the problems I have had in helping others is that we have been brought up to believe that only medications cure and it is hard for us to understand that nutrition is the solution to many of our ailments. I understood a long time ago that we are what we eat, but I did not know the correct way. Thanks to Uncle Frank I learned and continue to learn about this wonderful subject of metabolism."

-A. Durán

"I started my dietary change this year with the help of a friend and a nutritionist who motivated me to do it. Two weeks after starting my change, I happened to come across one of your videos that talked about the harm that microwaves cause in our metabolism. I remember watching a lot of your videos that day, and from then on, my life changed. With all your knowledge, your advice and help, here I am getting my metabolism back and living to the fullest. No more doctor visits... and I am 50 pounds lighter and several sizes smaller and all thanks to God who put me on the path to find your wonderful program!!! May God continue to bless you and fill you with years. Thank you, a thousand times over!

-J. Castro

"Thank you for the guidance and for everything else. With the book The Power of Your Metabolism and with the YouTube videos of MetabolismoTV, I have learned a lot and managed to lose 75 pounds (34 kilos). I am very grateful for your help."

-C. Quesada

"I have searched a lot of information from different sources, but my husband was the first to learn about you, and he recommended your videos to me. He is a nurse, and health is a very important topic. Since then, I have listened to your advice about rice and the 3x1 Diet and 2x1 Diet. I am one of those people that rice makes me fat even when looking at it. I used to be a size 16 to 18 and now I am an 8 to 10. I used to weigh 188 pounds (85 kilos), and today I weigh 153 pounds (69 kilos). A thousand thanks Frank."

-S. De La Cruz

"I live in Zihuatanejo Gro. Mexico. At the beginning of 2016 I was given a diagnosis that shook my life. I started with chronic pain in my arms, chest, and neck. I consulted many physicians, and they gave me anti-inflammatory medications, painkillers, cholesterol medications, relaxants and it went down, but it did not go away. I was diagnosed with breast cancer and had a very difficult time. This led my husband to search for information and he found Frank Suárez's videos. Topics such as water, candida, cancer, and the immune system, etc. He would watch and watch the videos to inform himself, while I was doing other therapies. My husband started to become my therapist, he would watch a video and try it with me. The pain and discomfort disappeared and although the fibrosis is still present in my breast, I had an MRI, and it is not malignant. My husband joined your courses, and these are the results: in two months I lost 15 pounds (7 kilos), in four months I lost 31 pounds (14 kilos) and went from a size 11 to a 5. Thank you".

-D. Rojas

"I am writing to you because I want to thank you for your book The Power of Your Metabolism, I lost 33 pounds (15 kilos) in five months and one year later my weight is the same. It is not dieting; it is changing my diet and lifestyle forever. I am happy."

-Y. Llerena

"I was a part of your online Metabolism Advisor course and I want to express my appreciation for the valuable insights, which when put into practice can really improve one's health condition. I am diabetic and to my personal satisfaction, I have managed to get my diabetes under control. Managing levels from 84 mg/dl to 106mg/dl of blood glucose. Previously my biggest concern was being unable to lower levels that fluctuated between 140 to 170 even on an empty stomach. Thank you for sharing so much knowledge and greetings from Morelia Michoacan, Mexico."

- J. Garcia

"I came to NaturalSlim due to health conditions. I had high blood pressure and was taking medications. Also, my doctor diagnosed me with prediabetes because my blood sugar was too high. I had gained a lot of weight after my last pregnancy and was wearing a size 16. It was very difficult to get clothes that fit me, and I always felt tired. Now I am off blood pressure medication and my blood sugar is under control without medication. I'm already wearing a size 8 and I feel great."

-G. Garcia

"I wanted to tell you about the progress I am making thanks to the book The Power of Your Metabolism and MetabolismoTV's YouTube videos, where Mr. Frank Suárez shares his knowledge with us and informs us of the truth! I have never had so much information and in the didactic way he explains it. I have been applying what I learned for almost four months now, and I am very grateful because I have learned to have a different lifestyle than the one I had before I have never been that obese, but I no longer felt comfortable in my clothes, and I felt that I was already getting worse. In these short four months I feel more energetic, I sleep better, I went down two sizes, and I am very happy about it. Nothing better than having knowledge and applying it".

-L. Geraldine

"I was a horrible size 20. My children and acquaintances criticized me. Everyone thought my problem was that I ate too much. But I learned that my problem was that I had a slow metabolism and a thyroid condition that my doctors had missed because it did not show up in my lab tests. Learning about metabolism allowed me to get the medical help I needed. By getting that help and improving my habits and lifestyle I was able to get down to my current size, size 8."

-S. Rodriguez

"I just want to thank you for educating me on the subject of metabolism, and by putting the 3x1 Diet into practice, my glucose levels have gone down; my A1c from 6.5 to 5.6. Also, as of today I have lost 68 pounds (31 kilos) from a size 28, I am down to a size 18 and I am continuing with my new lifestyle. Thank you, Frank, for helping me."

-I. Rivera

"I want you to know that your advice has helped me a lot. I bought your book The Power of Your Metabolism and I have done very well. In one year, I have managed to go down from a size 20 to a size 10. Thank you for your help."

-M. Sanchez

Ultra-Powerful Metabolism

A practical and personalized guide
of the principles that work to lose weight,
regain energy, improve health and maintain it.

Disclaimer:
This book, *Ultra Powerful Metabolism*, has been written as a source of information only. The information contained in this book should never be considered as substitute information for the recommendations of your qualified health care professional or physician. You should always consult with your physician before beginning any diet regimen, exercise, or other health-related program. The author, Frank Suárez, is someone who overcame his own obesity, he is not a doctor, dietitian, or nutritionist. He is an obesity and metabolism specialist in his own merit. The information provided in this book is based on recommendations that for over 20 years have proven successful for people seeking his help to lose weight and regain their metabolism. We have made reasonable efforts to ensure that all the information described here is accurate. Most of the information contained herein is based on the experiences gained from working with thousands of people on the NaturalSlim system (www.NaturalSlim.com). **You are cautioned against discontinuing or altering the dosage of prescription medications, changing your nutritional regimen, or use natural supplements without first consulting your physician.**

Ultra-Powerful Metabolism
© Copyright 2018-2022, All Rights Reserved by Frank Suárez, Manuscript and Cover Page

First English Edition: August 2022

Metabolic Press
262 Piñero Avenue, San Juan Puerto Rico 00918-4004

Cover design and illustration: Jocelyn Ramos & Idearte
English Translation: Idahlie Vázquez Delucca
Editing & Proofreading: Xiomara Acobes-Lozada
Printing: Panamericana Formas e Impresos S.A.

It is strictly forbidden, without the written authorization of the author of *Ultra-Powerful Metabolism*, under the sanctions established by law, the partial or total reproduction of this work by any means or procedure, including reprography and computer processing.

Trademarks: All trademarks of products or foods mentioned in this book are the property of their respective owners. The trademarks NaturalSlim, RelaxSlim®, 2x1 Diet®, 3x1 Diet® and others of products or services explained in this book are property of Metabolic Technology Center, Corp., and Frank Suárez.

Printed in Colombia / ISBN: 978-1-7321965-1-3

I dedicate this book to my followers at MetabolismoTV, to the members of the NaturalSlim System who trusted me to regain their health, and to all truth lovers.

Table Of Contents

- SUCCESS STORIES III
- INTRODUCTION XV
- AUTHOR'S NOTES XXI
- PATHWAY TO AN ULTRA-POWERFUL METABOLISM XXIII

KNOWLEDGE IS POWER 25
- THE BODY'S METABOLISM AND ITS ENEMIES 27
  - EXCESS SUGARS AND REFINED CARBOHYDRATES 31
  - STRESS AND ITS EFFECTS 36
  - METABOLISM ENEMY SUBSTANCES 38
    - POLYUNSATURATED OILS 39
    - MARGARINE 40
    - HIGH FRUCTOSE CORN SYRUP 41
    - ARTIFICIAL SWEETENER ASPARTAME 45
    - SOY 47
    - OTHER ENEMY SUBSTANCES 48
- CURRENT STATUS OF YOUR METABOLISM 51
- FALSE FACTS THAT AFFECT YOUR METABOLISM 61
  - THE HUMAN BODY IS A BOILER 62
  - FAT IS FATTENING 64
  - EGGS RAISE CHOLESTEROL 66
  - DRINKING A LOT OF WATER RAISES BLOOD PRESSURE 67
  - VITAMINS CAUSE HUNGER 68
  - THE BIG LIE OF LOSING WEIGHT 69

RESTORING THE METABOLISM 75
- THE RIGHT GOAL 77
- THE LIQUID OF LIFE 83
- WE ARE ALL DIFFERENT 95
  - THE TWO SIDES OF THE NERVOUS SYSTEM: EXCITED AND PASSIVE 106
  - HOW TO IDENTIFY YOUR TYPE OF NERVOUS SYSTEM 109
- THE 3X1 DIET TO RESTORE METABOLISM 119
  - EXPANDED LIST OF TYPE F FOODS - FATTENING 120
  - EXPANDED LIST OF TYPE S FOODS - SLIMMING 122
- THE RIGHT NUTRITION BASED ON YOUR TYPE OF NERVOUS SYSTEM 135
- HOW TO CALM THE NERVOUS SYSTEM 147
- REFINED CARBOHYDRATES DETOX 159
- SLEEP BETTER OR FAIL 167
- CANDIDA ALBICANS YEAST 177
- THE METABOLISM CONTROL CENTER 187
  - STEPS TO TAKE A TEMPERATURE AND IDENTIFY SUBCLINICAL HYPOTHYROIDISM 195
- THE AGGRESSOR FOODS 199
  - HEALTH-DESTROYING GLUCOSE SPIKES 210
  - THE RULES FOR FINDING AGGRESSOR FOODS 213
- THE HORMONAL BALANCE 219

- MOVEMENT IS LIFE 231
- INTERMITTENT FASTING TO HELP A STUCK METABOLISM 241
- THE ROAD TO RECOVERY 257
- PERSONAL PROGRAM FOR AN ULTRA-POWERFUL METABOLISM 263

REFERENCES AND ADDITIONAL AIDS 269

- NATURAL SUPPLEMENTS TO HELP YOUR METABOLISM 271
  - CANDIDA YEAST CLEANSING, CANDISEPTIC KIT 271
  - CONSTIPEND FOR CONSTIPATION 279
  - NATURAL PROGESTERONE FEMME BALANCE 281
  - DIGESTIVE ENZYMES HELPZYMES 284
  - POTASSIUM KADSORB 290
  - MAGNESIUM MAGICMAG 294
  - METABOIL 500 299
  - METABOLIC PROTEIN 303
    - FORMULA TO PREPARE THE METABOLIC PROTEIN SHAKE 306
  - METABOLIC VITAMINS 307
  - PASSIVOIL 311
  - RELAXSLIM SUPPLEMENT WITH ADAPTOGENS 315
  - STRESS DEFENDER FOR STRESS 319
  - TESTOSTERIN 321
- GLOSSARY: DEFINITIONS OF WORDS AND TERMS 325
- NATURALSLIM® LOCATIONS 347
  - NATURALSLIM® PUERTO RICO 347
  - NATURALSLIM® UNITED STATES 347
  - NATURALSLIM® PANAMA 347
  - NATURALSLIM® COSTA RICA 348
  - NATURALSLIM® COLOMBIA 348
  - NATURALSLIM® EUROPE 348
  - EL PODER DEL METABOLISMO CENTER CURAÇAO 348
- ADDITIONAL HELP SITES 349
  - METABOLISMOTV.COM 349
  - UNIMETAB.COM 349
  - PREGUNTALEAFRANK.COM 350
  - DIABETESTV 350
- ADDITIONAL HELP BOOKS 351
  - THE POWER OF YOUR METABOLISM 351
  - PROBLEM-FREE DIABETES 352
  - THE WAY TO HAPPINESS BOOKLET 353
- ADVISORS AND SPECIALISTS 355
- THEMATIC INDEX 359

INTRODUCTION

Frank Suárez and his work are a scientific and humanistic paradigm, a researcher who believes in science and what works, emphasizing the value and dignity of people. The founder of NaturalSlim has created a systematization of the principles of metabolism that contain a real technology that is revolutionizing the scientific community worldwide. His ability to observe the causes and solutions to problems is expressed in his direct communication, where with simple words he has helped hundreds of thousands of people who today thank, respect, and admire him. The restoration of metabolism has enriched the field of medicine, creating new capabilities in the care and prevention of diseases. Its results have been demonstrated and its potentialities are limitless, where there is hope for everyone at any age, being supported by the application of the latest research.

About three years ago, I was reviewing the latest information on thyroid cancer and discovered *The Power of Your Metabolism*, from that moment on I came in contact with this new world. After forty-one years of practicing my medical profession and working in hospital wards, intensive care and as a Professor of Internal Medicine, I gained this new knowledge. I took on the task of studying and researching everything related to its fundamental concepts that I applied with myself and my patients, obtaining excellent results. In my experience, personalizing each case by educating it, identifying the predominant nervous system, detoxifying the body, hydrating properly, cleaning the candida yeast, creating an active metabolism, avoiding the excessive use of refined carbohydrates, which contribute significantly to the growing epidemic of obesity, applying the 3x1 Diet, identifying and suppressing Aggressor Foods, performing physical exercises, solving hormonal imbalances, addressing mental and emotional states that are not pleasant, as well as identifying the type of stress and other measures related to lifestyle have been key in my work with my patients, convincing me that there is no disease that cannot be treated and improved, without exception, with the restoration of the metabolism from bronchial asthma to cancer.

In my medical records I have the tangible evidence of these results. Amazingly, patients recovered from ailments that they could not resolve, even with medications. I obtained significant advances in cases of diabetic neuropathy, I achieved the reduction of triglycerides in the blood without any medications eliminating the marketed statins; solving gastric reflux, gall bladder stones that were on their way to the operating room, depressive states, rebellious insomnia, solutions to migraines, ringing in the ears, sleep apnea, decreased libido and even sexual impotence, arterial hypertension, cardiovascular and cerebral disorders, hypothyroidism, diabetes mellitus, obesity; always ensuring that the updated, confirmed and published medical knowledge scientifically sustains the application and my medical conduct with my patients. I have consciously made it my mission to help patients and their families to better educate themselves, knowing the symptoms, avoiding, if possible, the prescription of medications, their toxicity, and complications in a simple, functional and above all effective way. My patients' satisfaction inspired me to continue deepening my knowledge until I reached the Doctorate in Metabolism. I recommend the reading and application of this book, *Ultra-Powerful Metabolism*.

As a Cuban, I actively participated in the construction of the health system of my country; proud and grateful for the ethical-professional training received from my teachers, I served as a physician in several countries, starting in Jamaica (1980-1981) through Algeria (2008-2009). I have lived this experience with integrity under difficult conditions, even in places where they had never seen a doctor. For seventeen years I directed, with different responsibilities, public health and achieved another specialty in health administration and the nomination of Doctor of Science awarded by the Academy of Sciences of Cuba. As a deputy in the Cuban Parliament, I assumed the responsibility of President of the Health Commission of the Latin American Parliament, visiting dozens of countries, seeing first-hand the health crisis we are facing and giving lectures, speaking at International Congresses. I have dedicated my life to the health field with the most humane profession that touches the soul of people.

Let us defend, let us take care of the legacy of the enormous achievement made by the author of this book who has put his knowledge at the service of humanity with humility, selflessness, and a vocation to help those in need, exposing his own experiences and overcoming multiple health conditions to become a hero of these times, and who continues with his work as a quixotic and with his dagger of truth, fighting against the current windmills.

Mexico, a hospitable country where I freely reside and where I currently work at the IMAGENUS Advanced Diagnostic Center, in my capacity as Chief of Staff of Check Up, needs, like other countries, this vision. It is an unavoidable duty to create a social movement that reaches all corners of the planet, that impacts on political will and constitutes a powerful force for the solution of our problems that fill our families with mourning. We hope that this technology is shared and perfected with scientific rigor and that we concentrate on helping people to confront physical difficulties, because it is a practical guide to build a world that needs to change, training them in the techniques and basic principles so that the person can apply it to health, not closing their eyes to pain, fighting to solve human suffering.

The biggest problem is that the trend is clear: the situation continues to worsen year after year. Raise awareness of the problem and its causes to protect ourselves and not become victims of ignorance. We all have a responsibility in one way or another. A new day can still arise for the men and women who need that hope. If the devoted work of Frank and his collaborators was multiplied by my humble work, inspired by his ethics, professionalism, and humanism, I wonder, how many doctors are currently unaware of these advances? Why do the programs of study for medicine students not incorporate these elements? If we know that it is proven science and that it respects recognized scientific research, some of them Medicine Nobel Prize winners, that the human body is related to everything; what a fertile field these advances in metabolism offer us for the application of the clinical method to diagnose with certainty, with the rigor of listening and observing the patient and understanding that health is not the absence of disease, that it is a biological-psychological-social balance and that we must understand that the body has to do with the mind and the being.

The way is paved for research work to be carried out with all that has been exposed and validated. How many patients would benefit from this? It is clear to me that a path is opening to find solutions to the current problems that plague humanity.

LET'S SAVE THIS LEGACY!

Dr. Ramon Crespo
Internist and Specialist
in Health Administration

Author's Notes

My purpose is to carry a message that serves to improve or recover energy, metabolism and overall health. The written message is communicated through words. Words have meanings that are not always known to all of us.

So, I do my best to avoid technical words or medical terms. Whenever I am forced to use a technical word, I make sure to also provide the definition of it so that the person does not lose interest in the subject and can understand it. Knowledge is power, but knowledge is acquired through the words of the language.

When I am forced to use a word that I think could be misunderstood, I provide the definition at the bottom of the page, and I also include it in the definitions that are in the GLOSSARY section at the end of the book. The idea is that you can locate new words in the glossary without having to use a medical or specialized dictionary. However, it is always a good idea to have a good dictionary handy because even a simple word of our common language that is not understood can take away your interest in what you are reading.

The same happens with the language. Many of the words used while speaking Spanish, my native language, are easier to understand in English than in Spanish.

Example: the human body produces a hormone that in Spanish is called "glucocorticosteroide" and is the hormone associated with stressful conditions. In English this hormone is called cortisol and naturally it is much easier to speak of cortisol than "glucocorticosteroide". Since my main goal is to get the message across to the readers, I choose to use the word that is easiest to understand and remember, with the permission of the language experts.

Pathway To An Ultra-Powerful Metabolism

The main purpose of this book is for you to establish the specific steps, in sequence, that you must take to restore your metabolism and achieve your goal, whether it is to slim down, improve your diabetes, or improve your overall health.

So, at the end of each chapter you will find a summary of the points discussed and one or more questions or exercises to perform. You can answer them here in the book or create your own guide on a notebook.

As you complete the exercises in each chapter, you will be creating your personalized program with the steps in order that will help you reach your goal.

I encourage you not to skip a single step of your Ultra-Powerful Metabolism Pathway. With the right knowledge and your determination to restore your metabolism, you will surely achieve your purpose.

I look forward to seeing you at the finish line,

Frank Suárez
Obesity Specialist,
Diabetes and Metabolism

Knowledge is Power

THE BODY'S METABOLISM AND ITS ENEMIES

Many people complain of having a "slow metabolism" because they find it difficult to slim down, gain weight too easily or feel deprived of energy. The word metabolism comes from the Greek *meta* meaning change or movement.

When we use the word *meta* in its sense of change, it is like when we speak of the word metamorphosis. Metamorphosis is a process of change of form. It is like when a caterpillar goes through a process of change and becomes a beautiful butterfly. Now, if we use the Greek word *meta* in its sense of movement it is like when we talk about a cancer[1] that is metastasizing. A cancer in metastasis is a cancer that is in movement, spreading throughout the body, already in its terminal stage. So, when we talk about metabolism we are talking about change or movement. So, what is metabolism? I offer you the following basic definition of metabolism to help you understand the topic:

metabolism: the sum of all the movements, actions and changes that occur in the body to transform food and nutrients into energy to survive.

---

[1] cancer: refers to a group of related diseases in which an uncontrolled process occurs in the division of the body's cells. Cancer begins to function independently from the body, spreads to other nearby tissues and can even cause death if left untreated.

There are many movements, processes, actions, and changes that the human body performs to survive: digestion [2], absorption, respiration, immune system (defense), circulation, elimination, etc. Each of these processes has one thing in common: movement. Movement always involves the use of energy. Without energy there is no movement. Your body's metabolism is what produces the energy that allows you to create all the movement, life, and health of your body.

The word *metabolism* has its origin in the Greek *meta* which means *movement*. Metabolism occurs within the cells[3] of the body and is the natural process your body uses to create the energy that keeps you alive and healthy. When a person experiences a slow metabolism, their body is lacking energy, so the person will also have a deficiency of internal movement which will cause them to put on weight easily, will have difficulty slimming down with diets and will most likely feel lacking energy to exercise.

When the metabolism is too slow, all the body's processes are also slow and this can be reflected in constipation, accumulation of toxics, poor circulation, many infections, poor digestion, overweight and obesity, diabetes, poor sleep quality and thyroid problems, among others. We could say that your body's metabolism is like

---

[2] digestion: is the natural process that allows the body to transform food into nutrients that can be used for the creation of energy produced by metabolism.

[3] cells: cells are the smallest parts of the body that contain life. In fact, cells, although extremely small, feed, digest and breathe just like you do. Your body's health depends on the health of the cells in your body.

the engine of your car. If the engine of your car is broken or not working properly, it will hardly go far or go at the right speed to help you reach your destination on time. Your car's performance will depend on how well you maintain it, the quality of the fuel and oils you use, among other things. Likewise, your body's metabolism performance will depend on how well you take care of it or how much you allow the enemies of metabolism to come into contact with your body.

Unfortunately, we have been harming our body's metabolism for decades. The wrong diet, contact with toxic substances and mostly the amount of false data out there, have led us into confusion with thousands of diets and "miracle remedies" that in the end only hurt us more.

However, even if it takes some time to restore metabolism, it is possible to do so and even break dependence on prescription medications for conditions such as diabetes[4], hypothyroidism[5], high cholesterol[6] and triglycerides [7], and even high blood pressure (hypertension[8]) medications. The secret is to first educate

---

[4] diabetes: diabetes is a condition characterized by having glucose (blood sugar) levels that are excessively high and harmful to the body's health.

[5] hypothyroidism: a condition in which the thyroid gland produces an insufficient amount of the hormones that control metabolism, body temperature, and body energy.

[6] cholesterol: cholesterol is a natural substance produced by the human body and by animals. Cholesterol is the main building material of many hormones, such as the estrogen hormone, which is the female hormone, and the testosterone hormone, which is the male hormone. All cells in the body contain cholesterol, except for the bone cells.

[7] triglycerides: triglycerides are fats that are produced in the liver. When someone is told by their doctor "you have high triglycerides" it means that the person has a lot of fat floating around in their blood, which is extremely dangerous for their health.

[8] hypertension: excessively high blood pressure. High blood pressure increases the likelihood of stroke, heart attack, heart failure, kidney disease or premature death.

yourself, have the knowledge of how your body works and manage everything that is affecting your metabolism.

It has been my mission, for decades, to research and bring to light those facts that are truly beneficial to our metabolism and overall health. After overcoming my own slow metabolism problem and helping hundreds of thousands of people in my NaturalSlim centers and through my books and my MetabolismoTV videos, I am absolutely certain that any metabolic condition can be improved if the right data, in the right sequence, is applied. Since truth always triumphs and I am totally committed to the truth, my purpose with this book is to take you through the proven steps that will unleash your metabolism and make it ultra-powerful; all built in the solid foundation of the RIGHT KNOWLEDGE.

In my books *The Power of Your Metabolism* and *Problem-Free Diabetes* I explain the things that affect the functioning of our body's metabolism the most. At the outset, it can be very confusing and can give the impression that EVERYTHING is harmful to us, when it is not. It is possible to improve our body's metabolism by managing the things that affect it and still lead a pleasurable lifestyle, without suffering or restrictions. Since to defeat the enemy, you must know it, let's briefly review some of the factors that slow down the metabolism.

Excess Sugars and Refined Carbohydrates[9]

There is nothing more enjoyable than eating a piece of freshly baked bread, a delicious plate of *gallo pinto* with fried *patacones*[10], some delicious *enchiladas*[11], a meat lasagna or spaghetti, a hamburger with fries, or some fried *alcapurrias* or *bacalaítos*[12]. And what about a chocolate cake with ice cream, or some donuts? All tasty foods that we cannot even think of living without. We are addicted to pizza, hamburgers, sandwiches, pastas, desserts, tubers[13], sugary soft drinks like Coca-Cola, milk, and the hundreds of thousands of versions of desserts that make us go crazy.

Sadly, the excess of all these refined carbohydrates and the overuse of sugar have not only fueled the obesity and overweight epidemic but affect the body's metabolism and overall health. The result, more and more people suffering from diabetes, hypothyroidism, and high triglycerides just to name a few of the health conditions that result from consuming excess refined carbohydrates.

---

[9] carbohydrates: carbohydrates cover a wide variety of foods such as bread, flour, pizza, tortillas, rice, potatoes, grains, sweets, sugar, and include vegetables (greens) and salads.
[10] "Gallo pinto" is the Costa Rican name for rice with beans and "patacones" are fried plantains, also known as "tostones" in the Caribbean.
[11] "Enchilada" is a Mexican dish made with corn tortillas bathed in a spicy sauce using chili peppers in its preparation. Depending on the style, the enchilada can be accompanied or filled with meats or cheese and with additional ingredients such as chopped or sliced fresh onion, lettuce, milk cream and cheese.
[12] "Alcapurrias" and "bacalaítos" are typical Puerto Rican fried foods. "Alcapurrias" are prepared with a mixture whose main ingredient is green plantain and some add "yautía", both grated. They are stuffed with meat and fried. "Bacalaítos" are made in a mixture of flour with spices and codfish that is fried in hot oil.
[13] tubers: tubers are edible roots, such as potato, sweet potato and cassava, among many others, which are carbohydrates and increase glucose (blood sugar).

The term carbohydrates encompass a wide variety of foods such as bread, flour, pizza, rice, potatoes, grains, sweets, sugar, and includes vegetables and salads. When we say refined carbohydrates, we refer to those carbohydrates that have been processed, cooked, ground, polished or refined in some way. This makes them much more absorbable and easily raises the body's glucose[14] levels. Almost all vegetables and salads (except for corn) are considered natural (unrefined) carbohydrates.

Although many of the natural carbohydrates are high in fiber [15], which does not harm us, within natural carbohydrates there are some carbohydrates that are very sweet tasting. Sweet carbohydrates can come from natural sources but the fact that they are sweet indicates that they are very high in sugar that can be converted to fat. Examples of sweet carbohydrates would be sweet fruits such as bananas, mango, pineapple, or raisins. There are also certain very sweet vegetables such as 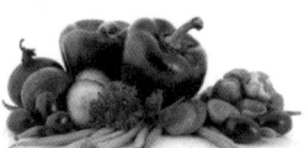 corn, carrots, beets, and tomatoes, which should be consumed very moderately, as they also easily turn into fat. There are some fruits that are not

---

[14] glucose: blood sugar that is the main fuel† and main nutrient of the body's cells.

† fuel: any material (gasoline, coal, etc.) capable of releasing energy when oxidized (it bonds with oxygen).

[15] fiber: is one of the components of carbohydrates. Although it is considered part of carbohydrates, it is a part that does not increase glucose and cannot make you fat. In fact, fiber helps reduce glucose absorption, thus helping you slim down. You could say that fiber is like a grain and does not provide any nutritional value, nor does it affect glucose.

excessively sweet such as strawberries and apples that are acceptable as natural carbohydrates.

Industrial processes to refine carbohydrates (wheat, rice, corn) are violent. Carbohydrates that are already refined are converted into wheat flour, corn flour, corn sweeteners, dehydrated potato, soy flour and other forms of refined carbohydrates. These foods are so refined, and their molecules[16] are already so small that the human body converts them into glucose quickly without much effort. Anything that increases glucose in the body too much will create excess body fat.

Note that more than 85% of diabetics are overweight. Diabetics are diabetics because their glucose levels are too high and because high glucose levels force the body to create body fat, over 85% of them are overweight. When we eat a donut (wheat flour with sugar) the body quickly converts it into a bunch of glucose and that creates excess glucose in the blood, which sets the scene for getting fat. That is the mechanics involved in the process of getting fat and one of the main factors that affect our metabolism.

The biggest problem of consuming refined carbohydrates in excess is that refined carbohydrates are addictive. People who are addicted to carbohydrates cannot control themselves. They eat the chocolates and

---

[16] molecules: the word molecule comes from the word moles which means mass. A molecule is a group of at least two atoms joined together. Molecules joined together form things and depending on the type of atoms that make up the molecule, it will be the type of element that we have. For example, fats are made up of carbon, hydrogen, and oxygen molecules.

hide the wrappers like evildoers. They are trapped in an addiction in the same way that the cigarette addict needs to smoke or the alcoholic needs to drink alcohol. Consuming these refined carbohydrates in abundance not only causes addiction, but it also causes a state of acidity in the body that slows down our metabolism. The excess of refined carbohydrates is converted into glucose once it has been digested. Some of the excess glucose is fermented inside the body and converted into lactic acid [17], which creates a state of acidity that reduces oxygen and metabolism.

Moreover, addiction to refined carbohydrates has a devastating effect on our mood, emotions, and excitement towards life. Excess refined carbohydrates cause sleepiness, tiredness, make people intolerant because they lack energy, and cause serious hormonal imbalances.

The way the body handles excess blood sugar produced by refined carbohydrates is that it secretes a lot of the hormone [18] insulin [19], which is the hormone that

---

[17] lactic acid: when blood glucose, which is a type of sugar, is fermented it is converted to lactic acid. Lactic acid, like all acids, is a substance that can create corrosion and damage to body tissues. For example, a person does physical exercise and then the muscles ache for several days. This happens due to the accumulation of lactic acid that is generated inside the body during exercise. It is called "lactic" because it was first discovered in milk products and that is why it comes from the word "lactic" (from milk).

[18] hormones: hormones are messenger substances in the body that carry commands that cause changes in the body. For example, the female hormone communicates messages to the body's cells that create feminine features (with breasts, no beard, more fat and less muscles), while the male testosterone hormone carries the opposite message of creating male bodies (no breasts, beard, less fat and more muscle).

[19] insulin: a very important hormone produced in the pancreas which allows glucose to be transported to the cells to be used as a source of energy for the human body. It is the hormone that allows the accumulation of fat in the body when there is an excess of glucose that is not

converts that excess glucose into fat. The problem is that INSULIN EXCESS interferes with the thyroid [20] gland [21] hormones. Doctors know that people with hypothyroidism also suffer from depression insomnia, constipation, difficulty slimming down and cold extremities, among other manifestations. This happens because the hormones produced by the thyroid gland control the entire metabolism of the body and its temperature. When the metabolism is affected, there is a hormonal imbalance that produces all these symptoms[22].

In fact, we should not restrict ourselves in eating a little piece of that bread or cake that we like so much. The point is to consume it in the right proportion that does not cause the hormonal and metabolic imbalance that comes from ingesting refined carbohydrates in excess.

---

used by the cells. Diabetics have problems related to this hormone and in some cases must inject it if their pancreas has already suffered damage and does not produce enough of it.

[20] thyroid: the thyroid gland is in the neck and is shaped like a butterfly with open wings. This gland produces the hormones that control the metabolism and the body temperature. When this gland fails in its production of hormones, it causes serious disruptions in the health and energy of the body.

[21] gland: is a body organ that has the capacity to produce substances that produce effects in other parts of the body.

[22] symptoms: a sign, indicator or signal from the body that warns of the existence of a health condition or disease.

STRESS AND ITS EFFECTS

Stress is a reaction that our mind and body have whenever they feel that survival is being threatened. Whether the threat is real or imagined, an unexpected noise or movement, accident, fall, blow, sudden change in temperature, concern with the present or the future, possible loss of something or a loved one, unexpected obstacle or problem, safety hazard or health problem or illness will cause a stress reaction. Stress is an instantaneous reaction that can be so violent that it can

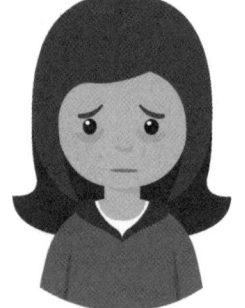

cause a heart attack. Usually, the reaction does not reach this point, but it does generate a state of GENERAL ALARM so strong that our entire hormonal and nervous system is affected. It is an effect that is cumulative. It is enough to observe how aged and deteriorated a person looks after the loss of a loved one to know that stress affects the whole body in a thousand and one ways.

Some people live in such a constant and continuous state of stress that they can no longer distinguish whether they are feeling stress or not. When stress is present on a routine basis, it is difficult for the person to become aware that he or she is going through a stressful life situation. For example, when a person experiences partner or family problems and must live with it day after day, he or she gets used to it and does not even realize that he or she is under stress.

In addition to the visible damage that stress causes to the body and health, there is a measurable factor: the hormonal factor. When there is stress, the body produces an excess of the cortisol[23] hormone. This hormone is called the stress hormone because it is always produced when a stressful situation arises.

Cortisol hormone is produced in the adrenal[24] glands which are located on top of each of our kidneys. This hormone is a vital[25] part of our body's alarm system. When the body feels in danger, say an annoying dog that wants to attack, the body produces the cortisol hormone which tells the liver to release stored glucose, because glucose is needed to have enough energy to fight or run and survive the threat.

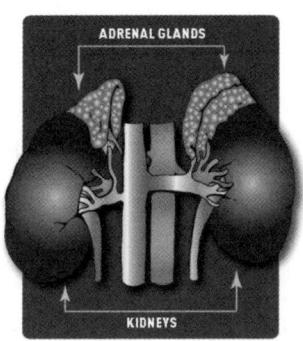

The problem is that when the source of stress is of short duration, like bad news, glucose levels increase due to cortisol, but when it is not consumed by the cells, it is converted to fat for storage. Glucose is the main source of energy for all the cells in our body, but when it is not used and is in excess, the body converts it into fat to store it as a source of energy for a future occasion. This is how

---

[23] cortisol: is a natural anti-inflammatory hormone produced by the human body in the adrenal glands. Cortisol is produced in the body under stressful conditions. It has an anti-inflammatory effect, but also increases body fat levels especially in the abdominal area.

[24] adrenals: on top of each of our two kidneys we have a gland that produces the adrenaline hormone which is a stress hormone. For this reason, they are called the adrenal glands. The adrenals also produce other hormones mainly the cortisol hormone which, among other things, accumulates fat in the body and is the reason why stress is fattening.

[25] vital: vital means that it is proper to life or that it is related to it. Vital means that it is essential for something to function.

stress produces an excess of glucose in the blood, through the action of the cortisol hormone, and that excess glucose ends up deposited in our waist, hips, and abdomen in the form of fat. Yes, stress is fattening.

It should be mentioned that the source of stress can be external or internal. By this I mean that also a situation of infection, internal disease of the body, even the consumption of foods that attack the body produces large amounts of cortisol because the body perceives the situation as something dangerous and reacts to it with an increase in the production of this hormone.

Metabolism is greatly affected by the cortisol hormone which is generated during times of stress. It is enough to know this to realize that our lifestyle is related to the condition of our metabolism and overall health.

Metabolism Enemy Substances

As we already know, everything we consume influences our body. Many times, the things we commonly consume can be the most harmful. Our processed foods have preservatives, colorants and ingredients that can cause hormonal imbalances and affect our health. This is the case of the substances below.

Polyunsaturated Oils[26]

These are oils such as corn oil, soy oil, canola oil, sunflower oil or what we know as vegetable oil. The problem with these types of oils is that, due to their molecular composition, they oxidize (rot) and affects the thyroid gland's performance. In fact, modern science[27] has recently discovered that canola oil specifically is extremely harmful and toxic to the thyroid and to health.

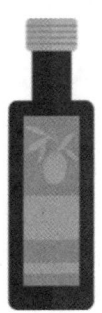

So, I recommend that for preparing foods that do not require frying, i.e., for your salads or sautéing your food, use olive oil. Olive oil is not recommended for frying as it does not withstand much heat. To fry your foods, use coconut oil, which also helps to increase your metabolism or use avocado oil.

Avocado oil should be the one that is cold extracted because this technique really gets the beneficial nutrients contained in the avocado such as all its antioxidants and Vitamin E[28]. In fact, avocado oil is extremely beneficial. It helps break down abdominal fat and can penetrate all the

---

[26] polyunsaturated oils: oils and fats are made up of molecules composed of carbon, hydrogen, and oxygen atoms. Polyunsaturated oils contain a large amount of carbon atoms that are not bonded to hydrogen atoms and therefore react to oxygen and can oxidize or rot. These are oils like corn oil, vegetable oil, sunflower oil, etc.

[27] science: the word science comes from the Latin *scientia* which means "knowledge". Science is an ordered system of structured knowledge that studies, investigates, and interprets natural, social, and artificial phenomena. Scientific knowledge is obtained through observations and experimentation.

[28] vitamins: vitamins are essential compounds for life and ingesting them in a balanced way and in essential doses promotes the correct functioning of the body. Most essential vitamins cannot be produced by the body, so the only way to obtain them is through the intake of foods that contain them. Vitamins are nutrients that together with other nutritional elements make all body processes take place.

way to the inside of the cells and helps rebuild them, plus it promotes the absorption of Vitamin B12, among other things. To learn more about oils that affect metabolism, I invite you to watch Episodes #1119 and #1275 on MetabolismoTV.

MARGARINE

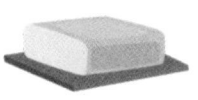

For decades we have been bombarded by the media about the dangers of cholesterol, to sell us cholesterol-free products. From this campaign came the idea of substituting cow's butter, which contains cholesterol, with the fat called margarine. However, margarine is not the healthy alternative that we are being sold.

All types of margarine have a high content of trans-fatty acids. Trans-fatty acids are fat molecules that have been damaged and deformed by the process of changing polyunsaturated oils (corn, soy, sunflower, vegetables) from their liquid state to a solid state and thus making margarine. This process of converting oil into solid fat is called hydrogenation and is carried out by heating the oil to high temperatures while applying electric current and pumping hydrogen gas into it.

Because of this, the molecules of the trans-fatty oils have lost their normal molecular shape and have become deformed. So, the body treats them as if they were toxic because it does not recognize them as edible and cannot use them for sustenance. After this whole process, the resulting fat, i.e., margarine, is of a white color that is not at all appetizing. So, margarine manufacturers add yellow coloring #5, to make it look like butter and make us want to eat it. The trans-fatty acids contained in margarine are very harmful to health and reduce metabolism.

Contrary to what the margarine consuming public is led to believe, there are several studies that show that the use of margarine increases cholesterol and increases the risk of heart problems. If you want to increase your metabolism and slim down, you should avoid margarine. Butter on the other hand, is a saturated fat that contains cholesterol, but it is a fat that the body can use naturally and does not contain trans-fatty acids that are harmful to our health. Butter is yellow because the cow and the creation decided so, it has no artificial colors. Butter will help you slim down; margarine will affect your metabolism.

HIGH FRUCTOSE CORN SYRUP

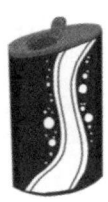

Scientific research indicates that fructose is much more harmful than regular sugar. The increase in national and international consumption of fructose corresponds exactly to the international increase in obesity and diabetes. The only organ[29] in the body that can use fructose is the LIVER, which

---

[29] organ: an organ is a grouping of cells that form tissues that work together in coordination to achieve some vital function of the body. Examples of some organs are the stomach, liver, lungs, and heart.

transforms fructose into URIC ACID[30], which is the cause of arthritis, gout[31], high triglycerides (fat) and several other inflammatory substances that begin to damage the walls of the arteries [32] and kidneys. Researchers at Duke University in North Carolina discovered that fructose consumption is the main cause of fatty liver, which then creates INSULIN RESISTANCE, which eventually ends up in a patient having to INJECT INSULIN and will become a permanent customer of one of only three insulin producers in the world: Eli Lilly, Novo Nordisk and Sanofi-Aventis.

In my book *Problem-Free Diabetes,* I mention the dozens of scientific studies that have proven the gigantic damage that fructose and high fructose corn syrup do to our bodies. High fructose corn syrup is a liquid sweetener[33] created from corn starch[34]. The vast majority of "natural juices" sold in supermarkets and the fruit juices that parents put in their children's snacks are sweetened with "High Fructose Corn Syrup", as you can read on the labels. In addition to its high fructose content, most of the

---

[30] uric acid: is an acid produced by the liver, muscles, intestines, and kidneys when processing purines. If the liver has lost its ability to detoxify the body and eliminate uric acid then diseases such as gout occur, due to over-accumulation of uric acid in the body.

[31] gout: gout is a disease caused by an accumulation of uric acid crystals in different parts of the body, especially in the big toes, soft tissues, and kidneys. It is a type of arthritis attack that causes intense pain and redness that is especially aggravated at night.

[32] arteries: these are the vessels or passages through which blood leaves the heart and reaches all parts of the body. They are the equivalent of what would be the body's pipeline through which the blood circulates.

[33] sweetener: a sweetener is any substance, natural or artificial, that provides a sweet taste to a food or product. Sugar and honey are sweeteners of natural origin, while sucralose or aspartame are sweeteners of artificial origin.

[34] starch: starches are molecules composed of simple sugars which are easily converted by the body into glucose. Carbohydrates that are starches such as potato, or sweet potato among others, are composed of starch. Rice is also a starch.

corn from which it is extracted and which we consume has been genetically modified[35], making it even more harmful.

Sadly, even with the existence of so many clinical studies demonstrating the harm that high fructose corn syrup does to our body and our metabolism, people with diabetes and the general public continue to be advised to consume products sweetened with high fructose corn syrup such as fruit juices, cookies, yogurt, ketchup, jellies, breads, cereal bars, canned pastas, canned vegetables, canned dressings, jelly, breads, cereal bars, canned pasta, canned vegetables, canned salad dressings, and canned fruit juices, among hundreds of other products.

If you look at the supermarket shelves you will see that they are full of products that claim to be "suitable for diabetics", or that are "fat free", "low in calories[36]" and "sugar free" (because they do not consider fructose as

---

[35] genetically modified: a genetically modified organism (abbreviated GMO) is a plant, animal, fungi, or bacteria to which certain genes† have been added by genetic engineering to produce certain traits or characteristics. In the case of corn, it is a corn plant whose genetic material has been artificially altered using genetic engineering techniques.

† genes: genes are microscopic markers that all body cells contain and serve to determine the traits that a living organism (person, plant, fungi, bacteria, etc.) will inherit because they transmit hereditary factors from one generation to the next. If, for example, mom and dad had green eyes there would be a strong possibility that a child of theirs would inherit the trait of green eyes. Genes transmit traits from parents to their children. Plants also have genes that pass on their characteristics and traits to their offspring.

[36] calories: the term calorie comes from French, which in turn originated from Latin "calor". In fact, a calorie is a measure of heat. It was a term created by French professor Nicholas Clément around 1819, to describe and calculate the conversion of the energy contained in coal when burned inside a boiler, to heat water to the point of converting it into steam to move a train engine. Although the term calorie originated in the physics of steam engines, the American chemist Wilbur Olin Atwater found and used it for the first time in 1875 in connection with his studies on nutrition and human metabolism. Atwater was the first to create the tables of nutritional values of foods and since then the term calorie went from measuring the energy of a steam boiler to measuring the energy that a food could supply to the human body.

sugar) that are sweetened with fructose in the form of high fructose corn syrup. It has even been said that fructose is better to sweeten your coffee, because as a "natural fruit sugar" it does less harm than other sweeteners. They may even recommend fructose from natural sources such as agave or coconut nectar and the truth is that they are very high in sugar. They are simply killing us with these recommendations.

Although fructose in high amounts, as used in soft drinks or to sweeten fruit juices, is very harmful, we will not go to the illogical extreme of confusing fructose with any known poison or toxin, such as aluminum and mercury metals, which need to be avoided in any dose no matter how small. Fructose can become a poison or be toxic to your body only if you abuse its consumption.

Fructose is part of vegetables as well as fruits. In general, it could be said that vegetables contain very little fructose and that fruits contain more. Fructose in small amounts, as with vegetables, may not be harmful. Fruits that are lower in fructose are fruits such as strawberries and apples. Try to avoid sweeter fruits such as mango, pineapple, and banana (in other countries it is called plantain, banana, cambur). We will not start now an illogical campaign to eliminate everything with fructose, because it is not necessary. It is the excesses that do harm and that is what we must avoid, the excesses.

ARTIFICIAL SWEETENER ASPARTAME

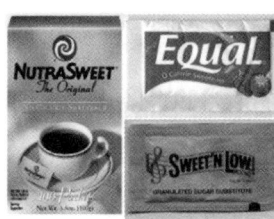

Most carbonated diet soft drinks are sweetened with aspartame. It is also sold as a sweetener for home or restaurant use under the brand names NutraSweet or Equal. This sweetener (sugar substitute) causes more than 75% of all annual adverse reaction reports received by the U.S. FDA regulatory agency.

Many of the reactions to aspartame are very serious, including cases of seizures, resulting in death. Other manifestations of adverse effects produced by aspartame are: migraines, headaches, dizziness, numbness of the extremities, weight gain, rash, depression, fatigue, irritability, tachycardia (rapid and uneven heartbeat), insomnia, vision problems, hearing loss, heart palpitations, breathing difficulties, anxiety attacks, loss of taste, vertigo, memory loss and joint pains. However, aspartame continues to be used in the market as if nothing is happening.

Most diet sodas are sweetened with aspartame. But besides this fact, you should know that drinking diet soda makes you FAT. There was a study in which Dr. Helen Hazuda from the University of Texas participated, in which it was clearly shown that diet soda is fattening. This researcher says, regarding the results of this study on diet sodas that "they may be calorie free, but they are not consequence free".

The researchers tracked the measurements and followed 474 people who drank diet soda for nine and a half years. They found that the diet soda drinkers had increased waist circumference by 70% over those years, versus those who did not drink diet soda. In fact, those who consumed at least two diet sodas per day had increases in waist circumference 500% greater than those who did not drink diet soda. These diet sodas are fattening, not only because many of them are sweetened with aspartame, but also because of their phosphoric acid[37] content, which removes oxygen from the body and slows down metabolism.

To sweeten your beverages and meals I recommend stevia, which comes from a natural source and does not affect your metabolism. You can use sucralose for baking, but I always recommend that you go for natural solutions.

---

[37] phosphoric acid: a type of acid contained in all soft drinks (including diet soft drinks) such as Coca-Cola and others, which destroys oxygen in the body and slows metabolism. The phosphoric acid in soft drinks is what causes the "little pins on the tongue sensation" that carbonated soft drinks cause.

Soy

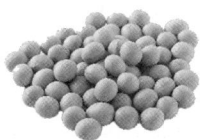

Soy was not edible until China discovered the process of fermenting them. Unfermented soy cannot be consumed because they have their own natural enzyme that makes them very difficult for humans to digest. The fermentation process makes it edible, but this does not mean that it is beneficial to our body.

Soy has a high content of phytic acid, which is a substance that blocks the absorption of essential minerals[38] such as calcium, magnesium, copper, iron[39] and especially the mineral zinc, which has a lot to do with protecting the immune system, with improving sexual function in men and with preventing prostate cancer. Zinc deficiency also causes depression and INSULIN RESISTANCE which leads to fattening and uncontrolled diabetes.

Soy also contains goitrogens [40], which are substances that block the function of the thyroid gland. Soy consumption forces the body to produce more TSH

---

[38] minerals: minerals are very important elements for health since, they help in the creation of different hormones, among other things, . Minerals are found in vegetables, salads and soil. Some minerals are magnesium, potassium, and iron.

[39] iron: is an important mineral that the body needs to produce hemoglobin, a substance in the blood that carries oxygen from the lungs to tissues throughout the body. Iron is also an important part of many other proteins and enzymes that the body needs for growth and development. Blood is red because of its iron mineral content.

[40] goitrogens: are natural or chemical substances that have been demonstrated they suppress the function of the thyroid gland. Anything that suppresses thyroid gland function reduces metabolism. Some natural goitrogens are contained in soy. The fluoride in toothpaste is also a goitrogen that reduces thyroid hormone production.

hormone, which is the hormone the brain [41] produces when it needs the thyroid gland to produce more thyroid hormone. The way to detect that a person has hypothyroidism is to look at their TSH hormone levels. If they are found to be too high, then you know that the person has an affected thyroid and is suffering from hypothyroidism.

The goitrogens contained in soy are not good for the metabolism. They directly affect the thyroid gland, which causes depression, obesity, fatigue, hair loss, insomnia, cold extremities, loss of interest in sexual activity and uncontrolled diabetes. Therefore, I recommend that you avoid consuming soy products, including soy milk, so that it does not affect your thyroid functions, which is the gland that controls the body's metabolism.

OTHER ENEMY SUBSTANCES

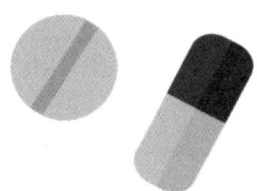

There are other substances that affect the body's metabolism, of which I have spoken extensively in my previous books. Substances such as fluoride, which has come to be used to treat people with hyperthyroidism[42] to slow down the thyroid gland's function; antidepressant medications,

---

[41] brain: is the part of the nervous system where our thoughts, perceptions (seeing, smelling, tasting, hearing) and emotions cause changes in all the functions of all the other parts of the body. The brain also generates the electrical impulses that control involuntary movements, or autonomous movements, such as breathing, heart rate, digestion, and others.

[42] hyperthyroidism: is a condition in which the thyroid gland produces an excess of thyroid hormones. This causes weight loss, palpitations, high blood pressure, insomnia, and panic attacks among others.

which increases the risk of developing the so-called metabolic syndrome [43], makes you fat and, ironically, causes depression, because it directly affects the thyroid; and acetaminophen[44] medication or paracetamol, which directly affects the liver and increases the risk of breast cancer. You can see more information about these substances in Episodes #1387, #1146 and #1303 of MetabolismoTV.

Also there are other factors that affect metabolism such as dehydration, the wrong nutrition for our type of nervous system, problems with the thyroid gland, digestion problems, fungal infections and the consumption of foods that are aggressors to our body, among other things that we will be seeing more in detail in this book, with which I aim to give you all the tools so you can really restore your metabolism and make it an ultra-powerful one.

Pathway to an Ultra-Powerful Metabolism

∞ Factors that reduce metabolism
- The excess consumption of sugars and refined carbohydrates.

---

[43] metabolic syndrome: when you suffer from insulin resistance, abdominal obesity, high triglycerides and hypertension (high blood pressure) at the same time.

[44] acetaminophen: acetaminophen, also known in other countries as paracetamol, is a widely used analgesic. Analgesic means pain reliever and is used for headaches, muscle aches, fever, sinus infections and sore throat. It is sold under different brand names such as Tylenol, Panadol, Mapap, Ofrimev, Feverall, Acephen and "Mejoralito", among others. In addition to these products, acetaminophen is contained in more than six hundred other products as part of the formulation of many, many other medications.

- The excess of emotional and internal stress of the body.
- The consumption of enemy substances to the metabolism such as:
    - polyunsaturated oils
    - trans-fatty acids -> margarine
    - high fructose corn syrup
    - artificial sweetener aspartame
    - soy
    - fluoride
    - antidepressant medications and acetaminophen

👓 Answer the following questions

1. To which factors that reduce metabolism have you been exposed? For how long?

2. What decisions have you made and what actions will you take after learning about the factors that reduce your metabolism?

Current Status of Your Metabolism

The human body is a perfect creation. At birth, our internal systems come ready to do their job and everything runs the way it should. A baby's metabolism is at its optimum performance, making sure that all the movements necessary for life are constantly occurring.

As we grow older and reach maturity, we gradually begin to lose the power of our metabolism as we age, and the body's movements slow down. Despite this, we can help our body to function at its highest capacity according to its age and have an ultra-powerful metabolism.

Our body carries out processes all the time to ensure our survival and well-being. It makes sure we breathe in the oxygen we need. It absorbs the nutrients our cells need to function. It filters toxins that enter the body through our liver and even has a sewage system, called the lymphatic system, through which cellular wastes, toxics and fat that need to be eliminated from the body flow, so we do not get sick. In addition, it has a defense system against diseases, viruses and bacteria and even collects the excess sugar in our blood and converts it into fat to prevent damage to our organs or to prevent us from going blind. There is no doubt about the complexity and extraordinary nature of the human body.

Now, you might ask yourself, if the human body is so well built, why I cannot slim down or suffer from diseases? Why do I have such a slow metabolism? The answer is very simple: we have been abusing our body for too long, due to misinformation and lack of correct data, causing it internal stress, feeding it the wrong way and exposing it to actions and habits that affect its proper functioning. Inevitably there will come a time when the body will not be able to handle the metabolic imbalance in which it finds itself and will have unpleasant manifestations.

When the metabolism is affected, we begin to suffer from symptoms that gradually worsen, until they develop into more serious medical conditions such as diabetes, hypothyroidism, high cholesterol and triglycerides and hypertension, among others. It starts with some fatigue or continuous tiredness; lack of energy to do the chores of the day or even to play with our children. We begin to have a poor quality of sleep and to wake up tired and without strength; to suffer from insomnia or to wake up many times during the night. It also happens that it becomes more and more difficult to slim down and even if we eat little, we put on a lot of weight.

Thus, gradually our system worsens, until we end up suffering from one or more of the following health conditions:

CURRENT STATUS OF YOUR METABOLISM

- ☐ cardiac arrhythmia
- ☐ arthritis[45]
- ☐ high cholesterol
- ☐ depression
- ☐ diabetes
- ☐ diverticulum[46]
- ☐ back pain
- ☐ autoimmune diseases[47]
- ☐ stomach gases / indigestion
- ☐ hemorrhoids
- ☐ hypoglycemia[48]
- ☐ hypothyroidism
- ☐ insomnia
- ☐ poor circulation
- ☐ diabetic neuropathy[49]
- ☐ inability to exercise

---

[45] arthritis: the word arthritis is composed of "-itis" meaning inflammation and "arthros" meaning joint, which is a place where one bone meets another. Inflammation of the bone joints is called arthritis.

[46] diverticulum: is a pouch that forms in the wall of the intestine. When they become inflamed, they can produce a number of unpleasant and painful symptoms, known as diverticulitis.

[47] autoimmune: refers to a disease in which the body's defense system, which is the immune system, attacks and destroys its own cells. The cause of autoimmune diseases is unknown, but everything indicates that the body has suffered an extreme and stressful incident that has caused some kind of intolerance, or there is a toxin, food or substance, or some kind of virus that attacks it, which creates a state of confusion in the immune system, and it attacks itself, as if it were its own enemy.

[48] hypoglycemia: is an abnormal reduction in blood glucose levels, which can cause dizziness, headache, cold sweats, mental disorientation and even unconsciousness. In principle, the body's cells begin to die from starvation due to the lack of glucose, some die, and the nervous and hormonal systems go out of control. This occurs when the blood glucose drops too low (below 60 ml/dl), which can happen due to an overdose of insulin, going too many hours without eating or intolerance reactions to certain carbohydrates such as rice or sugar..

[49] diabetic neuropathy: a type of nerve damage that occurs in people who have diabetes. This damage makes it difficult for the nerves to carry messages to the brain and other parts of the body. A diabetic may lose sensation in his or her legs to the point that he or she cannot feel the pain of a steel nail being driven into the heel of a leg. Diabetic neuropathy is also the cause of loss of sexual potency in diabetic men and the cause of sexual frigidity in diabetic women. Amputations usually occur after the person has already begun to experience some degree of diabetic neuropathy.

- ☐ osteoporosis [50]
- ☐ intestinal or vaginal polyps [51]
- ☐ high blood pressure
- ☐ heart problems
- ☐ liver/kidney problems
- ☐ reflux / acidity[52]
- ☐ high triglycerides

We do not have to suffer from these conditions to do something for our body. We just need to avoid habits that can affect our metabolism. We already know that the excessive consumption of refined carbohydrates slows our metabolism, but they affect it even more when they are the main component in our breakfasts.

When our body sleeps at night our metabolism slows down because the body enters its "repair" stage. When we sleep, all basic body functions are reduced and even breathing is much slower than normal. To sleep it is necessary to reduce the body's metabolism and energy production.

When you wake up in the morning, you need to increase your body's energy production to wake up your metabolism. This is achieved by exercising or consuming

---

[50] osteoporosis: loss of bone proteins and minerals. As a result, the bone is less resistant and more fragile than normal and breaks relatively easily.

[51] polyps: a polyp is a small protrusion that can grow in different areas of our body such as the stomach, gallbladder, uterus, vagina, and intestines, among other areas. Most of these growths are benign, but in some cases, if they grow too large, they can cause intestinal obstruction.

[52] reflux - acidity when the stomach is irritated, and its acids begin to move up the esophagus (tube leading from the throat to the stomach). This causes burning, irritation, and inflammation of the esophagus.

food. Now, if your breakfast consists of some oatmeal or some corn or rice cream (carbohydrates), accompanied by some bread toast (carbohydrates) and orange juice (carbohydrates) and coffee with milk (more carbohydrates), rest assured that, in addition to starting your path to diabetes early in the morning, you will not be providing your body with the energy it needs to wake up. Having breakfast like this only gradually slows down your metabolism.

Similarly, having a big meal in the evening and then quickly going to sleep slows your metabolism. As previously mentioned, sleeping slows down all the body's functions as the body enters its repair state. If you eat too much and do not consume the energy from those foods before going to sleep, the body will have no choice but to process that excess energy into fat, which makes you fat and reduce your metabolism.

There is another quite common habit of starving oneself. Whether it is because of some miracle diet to slim down quickly that was recommended to them or because they have the wrong information, many people decide to starve themselves, thus affecting their metabolism. The body is alive, which is why it can adapt to anything.

The reason why counting calories (starvation) diets do not work is because the body feels the drastic reduction of food that these diets bring. Initially, the person starts to lose weight, but their main loss in the first two weeks is a loss of water. Then, the person continues the diet and begins to lose weight, but notices that with each passing week the weight loss is less and less, and their metabolism gets slower and slower.

What has been discovered about this is that the body learns and adapts to food reduction by reducing metabolism. The body interprets the reduction of food as a condition of shortage. Its solution to the shortage is to slow down the metabolism more and more by reducing the function of the thyroid gland. Calorie diets and starvation give the wrong message to the body. The message is that it must slow down the metabolism because if it doesn't, it will run out of food. Since the body is designed to survive, its response is to reduce the function of the thyroid gland, and thus the metabolism, to survive on less food. This is an adaptive reaction of the body.

If you want to strengthen your metabolism you need to follow a type of nutrition that provides the body with what it needs to maintain your metabolism with the energy it needs. It would be a type of nutrition such as the 3x1 Diet[53] that we will discuss later.

---

[53] 3x1 Diet: a dietary regimen for metabolism restoration that considers the different effects that each type of food can have on the body's hormonal system (e.g., the amount of insulin the pancreas needs to produce). In addition, the 3x1 Diet is individually adapted for each person considering their biological individuality and the reaction that their CENTRAL Nervous System will have according to whether their nervous system is predominantly PASSIVE or EXCITED. A special feature is that in the 3x1 Diet foods are categorized as Type S Foods (SLIMMING – Helps SUPPORT the control of diabetes) or Type F Foods (FATTENING – Act as a FOE (ENEMIES) for the control of diabetes). The 3x1 Diet® is a registered trademark by Frank Suárez in the United States, Mexico and other countries in Latin America and Europe.

In addition to over-consumption of refined carbohydrates and poor nutrition habits, not managing stress and anxiety and not sleeping contribute to an impaired metabolism. Believe it or not, sleeping well is extremely important. While we sleep, the body carries out its repair processes. If these processes are interrupted, so is the proper functioning of our system.

Sleeping well involves resting in deep sleep for a minimum of seven hours so that our body can really repair itself. If you get up two or three times a night to go to the bathroom or your sleep is exceptionally light and any sound wakes you up, you are not really resting. This poor way of resting not only makes you feel tired when you wake up in the morning, but it can even raise your blood glucose levels and thus prevent you from slimming down. It can also cause you to wake up feeling very annoyed or grumpy, as you barely have enough energy to function. This immediately contributes to the stress we experience daily.

After not having slept well, we decide to skip breakfast and just drink a coffee. We get to work and there are problems to solve all over the place and on top of that, our grumpy boss, who probably did not sleep well either, comes into our area and yells at us for something that went wrong. Then we get a call from the school because Johnnie got hurt playing at recess, and after leaving the clinic with the child, the traffic back home is heavy, full of annoyed people also loaded with stress. At this point we are already super tired from all the day's hustle and bustle and there is no energy to cook, so we decide to go to McDonald's and get something quick: hamburgers, fries, soda, and an ice cream with chocolate for dessert. A feast of refined carbohydrates that now causes internal and alarming stress to our body.

This seems a bit chaotic, but if we think about it, it is a common day in the lives of many people, only that we are so used to it that we do not even think of it as a "stressful day". Add to the previous example the various relationship or family problems that we may have and with which we must deal with every day. It is very difficult to survive stress. The good news is that there is hope and we can handle it all, but first we must identify what state our metabolism is currently in and then we can help it.

Pathway to an Ultra-Powerful Metabolism

∞ **We can identify how our metabolism is affected by observing the following:**
- What is our energy level.
- How much is our ability to handle external and internal body stress.
- How good is our sleep quality.
- How many health conditions we are suffering from.

∞ **Answer the following questions**
1. Describe your energy level. Do you get tired easily or become fatigued? Do you feel like you are

"dragging your body" or do not have the strength to start the day?

2. Describe your sleep quality. Do you get at least seven hours of uninterrupted sleep? Do you feel rested and energetic upon awakening?

3. Describe your ability to avoid stress.

4. Write in here all the health conditions you have from the list presented in this chapter. Add any other that you suffer from that are not listed here.

5. Describe now what is the current state of your metabolism.

6. What decision have you made and what actions will you take after discovering the current state of your metabolism?

FALSE FACTS THAT AFFECT YOUR METABOLISM

The misinformation and the false facts we find in the media regarding metabolism, diets and health are one of the main reasons why our general state of health continues to worsen. We are in the age of easy access to information, but we are getting sicker and sicker.

Being sick is a good business for pharmaceutical companies. For example, since 1966 there are studies that show that excess consumption of refined carbohydrates is the main cause of many diseases, such as inflammatory diseases, liver problems and diabetes, among many others. However, people are not told what they really need to do to regain their health.

If you suffer from high blood pressure, they prescribe you medications for hypertension, but they do not explain to you what kind of nutrition or regimen[54] you should follow to really get cured and 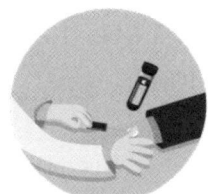 not have to take the medications forever. Things are this way because sick people are good business. A study by the investment accreditation institutions estimated that the annual drug market, for diabetes alone, will reach an

---

[54] regimen: a system or method of measuring and controlling the amount and type of food used in the diet.

estimated $58 billion in revenues by 2018. Do the math adding the hundreds of medications that exist for the rest of the diseases. Prevention is not a business for pharmaceutical companies. So, what we are encountering in the media is really a campaign of misinformation and false data that does not allow us to really improve, restore our metabolism and be healthy. A falsehood is a piece of information that is not true, that is wrong or that in some other way forces a person to make mistakes and be wrong. Let's look at some of them in detail.

THE HUMAN BODY IS A BOILER

Since the late 1800's it was argued that the only reason to gain weight was to consume more calories than we had expended. The term calories refer to the amount of energy a food can produce inside the body when ingested. If you look at the nutrition labels on foods, you will see that they tell you how many calories are in that food.

This type of classification on labels has been standard for decades and is based on the argument that people get fat because they are taking in much more energy (calories) than what your body consumes, so the body stores the excess calories as fat. So basically, if food consumption is controlled, based on its calorie count, then we avoid getting fat.

This statement is based on the comparison of our body with a coal boiler, like the one used in trains. If too much coal is added to the boiler, there comes a point when the "boiler gets fat", because too much coal was accumulated by not being able to be burned in its entirety. The same thing happens to our body. If this were correct, it would be enough to reduce the consumption of calories and we would not gain weight.

Although it is true that it is possible to put on weight by overeating, when this calorie theory was formulated, it did not take into consideration that the human body has life, so it reacts and adapts. So, this theory of calories has not given the expected results. We have been counting calories for decades and people have become 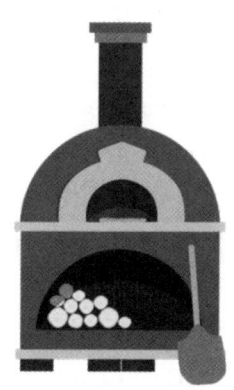 more and more fat. It has been recommended that you go on a 500, 1000, 1200 calories diet if you want to slim down. Besides the fact that you starve yourself and your body adapts to this by reducing your thyroid functions, these calorie-counting diets have very little protein (meats such as chicken, turkey, fish, beef, pork, etc.), as these are high in calories.

So, you go on a diet where you only eat salads, vegetables and potatoes, or rice, grains, or other carbohydrates, with very little protein. What you are doing is continuing to give your body a lot of carbohydrates and very little of what helps you slim down, which is protein.

Although you do start to lose weight at the beginning, what you lose is water and muscle weight that your body begins to consume in the absence of receiving more food. After a few weeks, your metabolism slows down, and you stop slimming down. So, our body is not a coal burning boiler and counting calories is not the solution to restore metabolism and slim down.

FAT IS FATTENING

We have been reducing fat consumption for decades. There are hundreds of fat-free or low-fat products, but obesity continues to rise. We have been sold the idea that fat produces more fat. This is a half-truth. It is true that the fat we consume may make us gain weight, but this is true only if the insulin hormone is present. Without the insulin hormone being present in the process of digesting food, fat cannot make us gain weight.

The way body fat is formed is as follows. You ingest food. Food is converted into glucose (blood sugar) so that it can be used as a source of energy. The amount of glucose generated depends on the type of food you eat. For example, proteins [55], because of their molecular composition, are converted into very little glucose; most

---

[55] proteins: proteins are foods that provide maximum energy to the body such as meats, seafood, eggs, cheeses, and proteins such as whey protein. Proteins are composed of amino acids† and do not cause the human body to produce a large amount of insulin as refined carbohydrates (bread, flour, pasta, sugar, etc.)

† amino acids: amino acids are the tiny components that make up proteins (meats, seafoods, cheeses, eggs, etc.). Depending on the types of amino acids in a protein is that you can differentiate between different types of proteins, such as between types of meats: pork, chicken, turkey, fish, etc.

vegetables, because they contain very little simple carbohydrates, are also converted into very little glucose. However, refined carbohydrates such as rice, *tortillas* or potatoes are converted into a lot of glucose.

After food has been converted into glucose, the pancreas [56] secretes the insulin hormone for it to transport the glucose to the cells and provide them with energy. However, if the amount of glucose is too much for the cells and the cells do not need it, then the insulin helps to convert the glucose into fat to store it and use it as a source of energy in the future.

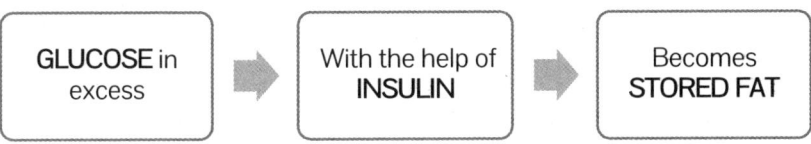

The reason why a diet high in refined carbohydrates causes weight gain, obesity and affects your metabolism is because no food group produces more glucose, more quickly, than refined carbohydrates. The greater the amount of glucose, the more the body is forced to produce more insulin.

Thus, fats are not the culprit. Fat will turn into more fat, only if you ingest it along with lots of refined carbohydrates. If you eat some fried *quesadillas*, you know that the fat from the oil will be picked up by insulin

---

[56] pancreas: is a gland about the size of your fist that is located right next to the stomach, toward the top of the abdomen. The pancreas produces hormones such as insulin and different enzymes to carbohydrates, proteins and fats.

along with the glucose that was produced from the carbohydrate in the *quesadilla* and will be stored in your body as fat. Enjoy your fried chicken, steak, or fried fish. Just do not combine it with a lot of refined carbohydrates.

EGGS RAISE CHOLESTEROL

All the confusion and false negative campaign that has existed since the 1960s against eggs, was finally intensified in 1984 when TIME Magazine published a study declaring eggs to be responsible for heart attacks because of their cholesterol content. In July 1999, a new study finally declared egg cholesterol innocent of causing harm to the body.

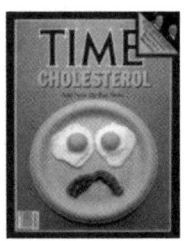

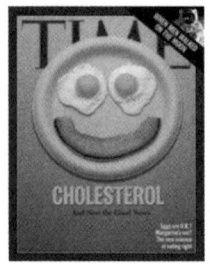

Eggs and their cholesterol content have been studied over the years with better and better news. Eggs have been found to reduce the risk of atherosclerosis[57] and stroke. It has also been proven that consuming three eggs a day causes good cholesterol (HDL) to rise to healthy levels and bad cholesterol (LDL) to drop or remain the same, when combining egg consumption with a low-carbohydrate diet. In short, eggs are a perfect protein, very beneficial, that combines magnificently with

---

[57] atherosclerosis: a condition in which the walls of the body's arteries (heart, brain, etc.) become inflamed, suffer damage and fill with a plaque of fat and calcium that clogs circulation. Arteriosclerosis or atherosclerosis hardens and stiffens the arteries, so they lose the flexibility to expand when the heart pumps and raises blood pressure. The arteries, in effect, also become blocked and that is what causes a heart attack or stroke.

almost any other food in the type of nutrition we recommend restoring your metabolism.

Drinking A Lot of Water Raises Blood Pressure

It is completely false that drinking water raises blood pressure. In fact, one of the most effective ways to lower blood pressure is to DRINK ENOUGH WATER EVERY DAY. This is such a simple solution that nutrition experts find it unrealistic.

65% of our body is water. Water is a vital fluid for life and for all body processes. If you do not drink the daily amount of water your body needs, all its processes are affected and, in effect, this also causes your blood pressure to rise. What happens is that, when dehydrated, the body increases the production of vasopressin hormone, which is an anti-diuretic hormone, that is, it prevents you from urinating or losing water in sweat or otherwise. Vasopressin does exactly that, it presses on the blood vessels to prevent you from losing more water. As the capillaries close to keep from losing water, it increases the body's blood pressure.

So, <u>not drinking water raises blood pressure</u>, while drinking enough water lowers blood pressure. In the chapter THE LIQUID OF LIFE we will see exactly how to determine how much water you need to drink daily, according to your body's specific needs.

In addition to dehydration, obesity is one of the main causes of hypertension. When a person is too obese, the excess fat in his or her body accumulates excessively on the walls of the arteries, thus reducing the space that is free for the blood to pass through. The arteries become clogged, making it difficult for the heart to pump blood to the different parts of the body. The heart reacts to this problem of blocked arteries by pumping harder, which causes high pressure.

VITAMINS CAUSE HUNGER

It is not true that vitamins make you hungry. What makes you hungry when taking vitamins are the SERIOUS DEFICIENCIES of vitamins and minerals that have accumulated in the body over many years of poor nutrition. If a person feels increased hunger when taking vitamins, it means that the body was so deficient in vitamins and minerals that the metabolism has been awakened and now the cells of the body, which are like little ovens, are asking for food to burn. If the person gets hungry it does not mean that he or she is going to gain weight. It only means that the metabolism is being activated and what should be done is to give food in the right way and never exceeding in the consumption of refined carbohydrates.

In fact, we must feed our body with good vitamins that are potent and that supply the amounts our body needs for proper functioning. Commercial vitamins, which in my book *The Power of Your Metabolism* I called "low potency", do not really supply the amounts of minerals and vitamins that our body needs. Supplement with good vitamins and you will see the change in your energy and improvement in your metabolism quickly.

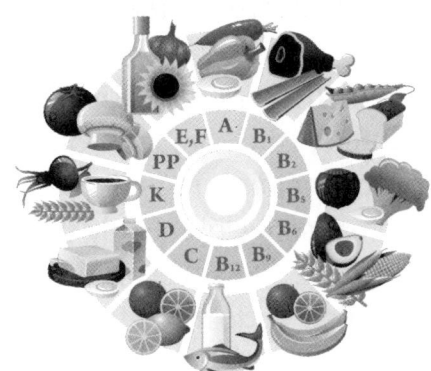

THE BIG LIE OF LOSING WEIGHT

If you suffer from obesity or excess weight, you should avoid falling into the big lie of "losing weight". The problem is not your body weight, the problem is the excess fat stored in your body, which is what is called obesity. Slimming down and losing weight are not the same thing.

When you are on a diet too low in calories or too low in fat your body starves. What happens internally when there is a shortage of food is that the body, in order to survive, increases the amount of cortisol hormones (stress hormone), to destroy a good part of the muscles of the body and give them as food to the cells, in order to sustain life. Much of the weight you lose on a diet that is too low in calories is not fat weight, it is muscle weight that was destroyed to feed the cells. What you really want to achieve is to **slim down** if you are overweight or obese and to control diabetes. This means **reducing body fat** without destroying the muscles, which means **you cannot starve yourself**.

In the twenty plus years of operating NaturalSlim centers, the biggest obstacle we have had is the **misconception** most people have that their goal should be to lose weight. Body weight is not a good measure of progress. However, measuring waist circumference is, because it clearly reflects the reduction in body fat. By restoring metabolism, the amount of energy produced by the body's cells is dramatically increased and stored fat begins to be consumed. This reduces fat throughout the body, but especially in the abdominal area.

If you are a lady with a size 24 pant size, who weighs about 260 pounds (118 kg), it does you no good to lose 40 pounds (18 kg) of weight and find that you are only down to a size 20. What you want is to **slim down** those 40 pounds but of **fat**. If you eliminate that amount of fat, rest assured that you will be modeling a slim size 10-12 figure

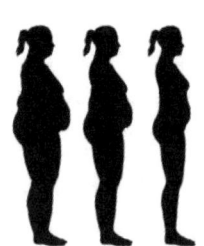

and you will feel full of energy. For sure your body weight will not reflect much change and you will drop to approximately 225 pounds, because as you eliminate fat you create more muscle mass and muscles are heavy.

Most people have a serious misunderstanding of fat. Fat is not a heavy substance. In fact, the lightest thing in the body is fat. What really weighs a lot in the body is water, muscle, and bone. Think of fat as a cushion (pillow) made from sponge. You can decorate the seats in your house with very large cushions filled with sponge, which take up a lot of space, yet they are very light; they are almost weightless. So is fat; it is very light, but it takes up a lot of space.

When a person does physical exercises muscle mass will increase and therefore the body weight will go up. But by exercising, the person is increasing muscle mass while reducing body fat and therefore will be heavier, but also slimmer and with less body fat.

So, what you want to do is increase your metabolism and become **slimmer**. Forget about the dammed weight! What good would it do to you to lose weight if your clothes got tighter and tighter? What you really want to watch is your size (clothing size) or your waist. You want the fat to go away, not the skin to hang off you like a bandage. Ignore the Big Lie of Losing Weight and start enjoying the slim figure and restored metabolism you deserve.

Pathway to an Ultra-Powerful Metabolism

👀 False facts that affect your metabolism
- Dieting by counting calories.
- Thinking that fat produces more fat. What is really fattening is the excess of refined carbohydrates.
- Thinking that eating eggs raises cholesterol. Eggs are a perfect protein, which helps the metabolism.
- Thinking that drinking water raises blood pressure. On the contrary, water is necessary to control hypertension.
- Malnourish the body by not taking vitamins, thinking that they will make the body hungry and fat.
- Believing the big lie that we are too heavy and that we must "lose weight". What we need to do is to **slim down** and reduce clothing sizes and body fat.

👀 Answer the following questions
1. Which of the of the false facts mentioned above have you heard before?

2. Which of these false facts have you practiced in your life? What have been the results?

3. What decision have you made and what actions will you take after discovering the truth about these false facts?

Restoring The Metabolism

THE RIGHT GOAL

Before you start applying the correct steps in sequence to restore your metabolism, know that the most important thing is to set the correct goal and not start with false expectations. What I mean by this is that by understanding how our body's metabolism works, we can set goals that are realistic about what we will achieve.

We found out that there are thousands of promises of "miracle pills" that will help you slim down "50 pounds (23 kilos) in one month". "Lose 30 pounds (14 kilos) in 30 days and pay only for the cost of food". "Use this wonderful machine and drop your waistline in two months". We are so bombarded, that little by little we make false expectations of what we can achieve in a short amount of time. Having the wrong goal will force you to fail.

The truth is that we have been damaging our metabolism for so long with the excessive consumption of refined carbohydrates (pizza, tacos, hamburgers, sandwiches, pastas, desserts, rice, potatoes, donuts, cakes, etc.) and without managing stress, and other things, we have affected the functioning of our body's metabolism. We cannot expect that all the damage we have caused will be solved in a few days.

Yes, by starting a metabolism restoration regimen you will begin to see changes quickly. But we must set our goal based on the right data. For example, if you are looking to slim down, it is most recommended that you lose one to three pounds of fat per week (.45 to 1.36 kilograms per week). Losing much more than this on a weekly basis will contribute to sagging skin that does will not have time to settle into place naturally.

The most important thing is not to set the wrong goal of "losing weight". As we have already explained, there is an important difference between losing weight, which can mean muscle or water loss and damages the body, and having the right **slimming** goal, which means **reducing body fat.** By slimming down using proper nutrition and hydration, the body gains muscle, and hydrates, which avoids permanent damage to the skin with stretch marks or sagging skin that makes it look bad, as happens with starvation diets.

Look at this photo with two men who have the same weight. They both weigh 200 pounds (90 kilograms).

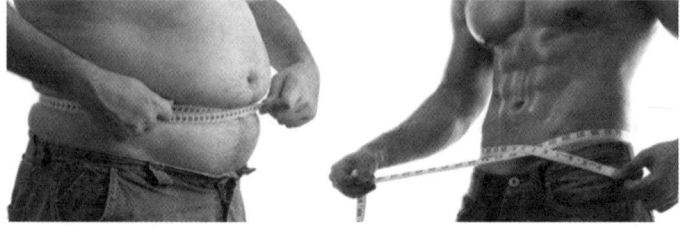

The one on the left **has a lot of fat** and the one on the right **has a lot of muscle and water.** The one on the left will have poor health and little energy and the one on the right will have good health and lots of energy. Although they both weigh 200 pounds, their bodies are very different.

When we want to restore our metabolism, the most important results and healthy goals should be:

1. **Reduce your clothing size** (waist measurement in men), which is what happens when <u>body fat is reduced.</u>
2. Increase your energy level.
3. Control your nervous system.
4. Improve your health state.

Remember that clothes do not lie, nor are they forgiving. If you are truly slimming down, it will be reflected in a leaner, more energetic body. To visually understand this topic, I recommend you watch Episode #500 on MetabolismoTV.

In case you have diabetes, in the book *Problem-Free Diabetes* I explain in detail how to achieve control of your diabetes, but as a summary, the additional goals for you would be:

1. Maintain glucose below the danger range, which is 130 mg/dl.
2. Make sure that glucose always remains within the normal range, which is between 70 mg/dl and 130 mg/dl.

3. Reduce inches (centimeters) from the waist and slim down.

Pathway to an Ultra-Powerful Metabolism

ᛆᛆ The correct goal
- It is important to establish the right goal and eliminate false expectations.
- The correct goals should be within the following:
    - reduce clothing size
    - increase energy levels
    - control the body's nervous system
    - improve general health status

ᛆᛆ Answer the following questions
1. Make a list of all the failed attempts you remember making in your life to slim down or improve your health. (Examples: Slimex100 pills, HCG drops, Adipex, grapefruit diet, nutritionist, Alli medications, counting calories, fat avoidance, exercise/walking, gyms, etc.).

2. Find in your mind what was your **Basic Purpose** behind all the previous efforts you made and ask yourself what was it that you wanted to achieve? What was the main reason that motivated you to invest effort or money in all the failed attempts? For example: *"to put on clothes that do not fit me", "to be able to wear size 4 clothes, like before I got married", "to look good for my partner", "to feel good when I look in the mirror", "to improve my diabetes", etc.).*

   Once you find it in your mind, write it down here.

3. Now the important question to ask yourself is, that basic purpose of yours, is it still something you would like to have? If the answer is yes, you have rehabilitated your basic purpose and you can now choose your correct goal. If the answer is NO, spend some time until you find out what your true personal basic purpose is in terms of metabolism, health, or slimming down, and write it down here.

4. Set your personal goal now in clothing size and health achievements.
   - My current clothing size or waist measurement is:

   - My goal in clothing size or waist measurement is:

   - My health goal is: (For example: "control my diabetes", "get my doctor to take me off my medications", "lower my cholesterol", "lower my triglycerides", "lower my blood pressure", "get a good night's sleep", "feel more energetic", etc.).

5. What decision have you made regarding your correct goals in restoring your metabolism?

THE LIQUID OF LIFE

Understand that without water, there is no life. All of us, before we are born, spend nine months floating in a lake of water, called the placenta, in our mothers' wombs. Without water and oxygen to breathe, there is neither life nor health.

The water molecule, when you see it drawn, looks like Mickey Mouse's [58] face with two ears. The chemical symbol for water is H2O. It means that the water molecule is composed of two hydrogen atoms[59] and one oxygen atom. Look at the water molecule and you will see that the oxygen atom is much larger (it is eight times larger in size) than the sum of the two small hydrogen atoms would be:

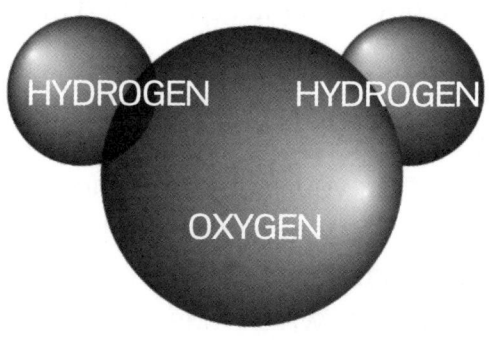

8 times bigger

---

[58] Mickey Mouse: fictional character of the Disney company, who has a round face and two smaller round ears.
[59] atoms: the atom is the smallest unit particle of matter or substance that can exist. Solid matter, food and substances are all composed of atoms that form them when they are joined together. The word atom comes from Greek and means "not divisible".

In other words, when you drink water, what you are primarily ingesting is **oxygen**. That oxygen is what provides the ability for your body's cells to breathe, thus restoring metabolism. Metabolism depends on the internal combustion[60] of cells, and that combustion is impossible without oxygen. Based on the molecular weight of the oxygen atom and the weight of the two small hydrogen atoms that make up water, it turns out that the water we consume is composed of 88% pure oxygen.

To create the energy in our body that allows us to move and live a healthy life we must restore our body's metabolism so the cells can do their work efficiently. The cells in our body are like little power plants. You have trillions of cells in your body, that is, millions, millions, millions, millions of cells that could produce energy. But when our metabolism is affected, it is as if a part of those cells, which are power plants, are turned off.

To restore metabolism and rehabilitate the energy production capacity of those cells that seem to be off, you must start by giving your body the amount of WATER it needs. When you feel you have a lot of energy and do not get tired easily, what has happened is that many of those cells were activated, which due to lack of water and adequate food, were shut down and therefore could not contribute with their energy. Restoring your metabolism is like turning on all the lights in a building that was partially dark and gloomy because it had too many lights

---

[60] combustion: energy-creating reaction of a combustion with oxygen.

off. Drinking enough water according to your body weight allows this to happen.

When your metabolism is working well you will feel you have a lot of energy and a desire to move your body. If your metabolism is deficient (slow metabolism) you will be "piggy backing" your body and sometimes feel like you are dragging it along. This happens because your body's cells are not producing enough energy, which happens, in large part, because your body does not have enough water to trigger the creation of cellular energy.

The body's metabolism occurs inside the cells, specifically in the mitochondria. The mitochondria are the part of the cell that functions as a small oven that produces energy. When you ingest food, the body breaks it down into very small particles that are transported into the cells. Then the mitochondria pick up those nutrients and mixes them with oxygen, generating combustion, which produces heat energy. That is why, when our metabolism is working well, we feel our body warm. That heat energy is a substance called adenosine triphosphate, or ATP for short. ATP is the body's internal chemical energy, which enables the movement we call "life".

The main characteristic of life is movement; dead things do not move. When you get your body cells to produce more ATP you will feel a lot of energy, you will not get tired easily, you will be able to slim down, your mind will work well and you will be able to learn, you will sleep well, and you will even be able to control diabetes if you suffer from it.

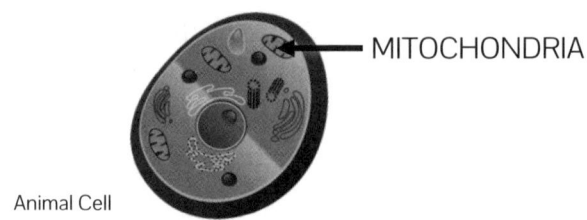

Animal Cell

One fascinating thing I found in scientific literature is that in 1970 it was discovered that water consumption (having good hydration) causes the ATP that produces the body's cells to multiply in its potential energy by almost ten times. So, ATP depends on your water intake to be activated to its full potential and provide your body with abundant energy. When ATP meets water and becomes hydrated, a reaction occurs that multiplies the energy of ATP.

The wonderful energy-creating properties that water produces inside the body's cells and that have a decisive influence on your metabolism, have been extensively studied by scientists over the last few years. Unfortunately, it is such an inexpensive solution to improve your health that it is not given much publicity.

Since I published my book *The Power of Your Metabolism*, I have made known the importance of sufficient water consumption in the process of restoring metabolism. People who suffer from slow metabolism put on weight too easily and slim down too slowly simply because their metabolism is not burning body fat; and one of the main causes of this is DEHYDRATION.

The formula we recommend to determine how much water your body needs to consume daily, which is the same formula we have been using successfully for over twenty years at NaturalSlim, is taken from the recommendations of Dr. Batmanghelidj. He is the author of the book *Your Body's Many Cries for Water*. Using this formula to calculate how much water to drink each day we have had excellent results with members of the NaturalSlim System, both in helping them slim down and in controlling diabetes. This formula takes into consideration that the larger a body is, the more water it needs, so the daily water requirement is calculated based on a person's body weight.

The formula is as follows when body weight is calculated in pounds:

> **BODY WEIGHT IN POUNDS divided by 16, equals how many 8 OUNCE GLASSES OF WATER you need to consume each day. Example: a person weighs 176 lb/16 = 11 glasses of water of 8 oz.**

When body weight is calculated in kilograms, we use the following:

> **BODY WEIGHT IN KILOGRAMS divided by 7, equals 250 MILILITER GLASSES OF WATER you need to consume each day. Example: a person weighs 84 kg/7 = 12 glasses of water of 250 ml.**

Whether calculating weight in pounds or kilograms, the formula always produces the same result. When the person slims down, thereby reducing their body weight and size, the calculation requires them to reduce proportionally based on their new weight.

The usual recommendation that we are accustomed to of "you should drink eight glasses of water a day" is not very logical because it does not consider the size of the body, which is what determines your need for daily water consumption. It is not the same to have a 160-pound body (73 kilos) that needs 10 glasses of water as it is to have a 240 pound body (109 kilos) that needs 15 glasses of water.

Something very important is that drinking other flavored liquids such as soft drinks, fruit juices, milk, coffee, tea, and flavored water, among others, <u>is not the same for the body as drinking water</u>. When a liquid has some flavor the sensors in the stomach wall detects that flavor and the body handles it as if it were food, producing hydrochloric acid [61] to digest it. Our interest is not to activate digestion, but to hydrate the body. So, what is recommended to restore the metabolism is to drink WATER, pure H2O without anything added and without any flavor.

People who are very dehydrated hate water and feel they can't tolerate it, so they try to drink any liquid that is flavored. But know that to really achieve an ultra-

---

[61] hydrochloric acid: acid produced by the stomach to help digest food.

powerful metabolism you must drink water. The body adapts to everything. At first it may even make you nauseous to drink water, because you have kept your body without water for so long that your body doesn't want it anymore. The key is not to despair and continue to give it water. By the third day you will crave water and your body will no longer ask for other liquids, because the ENERGY that water produces in your metabolism will have increased.

In addition to the fact that not drinking water reduces your body's energy production, not drinking water brings additional problems to the body. To survive without water, the body rations internally and leaves water available only for the exclusive use of vital organs. So, people who are dehydrated begin to have dry mouth and even lack of tears and sweat. Blood pressure rises, as capillaries close to avoid losing what little water the body has left.

In addition, dehydrated people begin to have problems of bad breath, because the body has a reduced capacity to eliminate its wastes due to the lack of water for urination and defecation. They also get swollen ankles in their legs, as the body tries to retain what little fluid it has. Being dehydrated also affects the kidneys' ability to do their job, so we must drink water to avoid damage to both the kidneys and the rest of our body's organs.

Another area that is greatly affected by lack of water is the functioning of the sexual organs. Dehydration aggravates sexual impotence in men and reduces sexual desire in women. A man's sexual system is a hydraulic system (working based on water pressure), which is what can create and maintain an erection. Men who are dehydrated have blood that is too thick, so it does not pass easily through the smaller capillaries in the penis. Human blood is 92% water and dehydrated people have blood that is too thick and does not flow as easily, which affects sexual function. In the case of women, if they do not stay well hydrated, they have problems with sexual activity because they begin to suffer from excessive vaginal dryness that makes sexual activity painful and undesirable.

Water is the liquid of life. This does not mean that you cannot consume other beverages if you do so in moderation. The "natural fruit juices" sold in stores are too high in sugar, as they are sweetened with high fructose corn syrup and are not really recommended. If you want to drink a natural, homemade fruit juice, you can enjoy it in small quantities and if you sweeten it with something extra, do it with stevia and not with sugar.

As for the use of coffee or tea, there is no problem in consuming them, if it is done in moderation (up to two to three cups per day). What you should avoid is drinking them with milk, sugar or honey. You should prefer to use substitutes low in refined carbohydrates such as milk cream (which is the fat in milk) or the product called "half and half", which is half milk and half cream. Now, remember that the caffeine contained in coffee and tea is a diuretic[62] it extracts water from the body and forces it to urinate. So, if you consume them, you must compensate for the water that the caffeine makes you lose so that you do not become dehydrated.

The consumption of alcoholic beverages, when done in small amounts, may be acceptable. But if you are one of those people who find it very difficult to control their alcohol consumption, it is best not to consume it at all, as you will not be able to moderate it. If you want to consume alcohol you should do so in moderation and without mixing it with sweet juices or soft drinks (Coca-Cola, 7Up, Pepsi, etc.) or with any other source of carbohydrates. A glass of red or white wine, a shot of whiskey, vodka, rum, tequila, or other alcohol with soda (carbonated mineral water), even a beer, would be tolerable. Sweet drinks and after-meal cordials[63] are too much sugar.

Alcoholic beverages are composed of very simple carbohydrates that are quickly converted into glucose and will make you fat, therefore their consumption should be extremely moderate. However, the main problem is that alcohol is a diuretic and dehydrates the body. You only need to look at how often people go to the bathroom to urinate while drinking alcohol to know this is true. If you plan to go to a social activity and you know you will be

---

[62] diuretic: a medication that works by extracting and reducing the volume of water in the human body to reduce blood pressure. When a diuretic is used, the person increases the volume of urine excretion and thus reduces the pressure.

[63] cordials: they are also known as digestive liqueurs. They are the alcoholic beverages that are drunk after eating to settle the stomach and have a good digestion. They are drinks such as brandy, cognac, and gins, among others.

drinking alcohol, make sure you have hydrated your body well before you go. You should do this to prevent the alcohol from drawing so much water out of your body that it dehydrates you and slows your metabolism. Then, while consuming alcohol, make sure you also drink water and then drink a lot more water to replace the loss.

Drinking water has many benefits: it restores your metabolism and gives you energy, helps you slim down, lowers blood pressure, aids in the elimination of toxins, helps with constipation and with the optimal functioning of all the organs of the body. It improves sexual activity, diabetes and even skin health. In short, consuming the amount of water your body needs daily is your first step to an Ultra-Powerful Metabolism.

Pathway to an Ultra-Powerful Metabolism

☞ Life depends on water and oxygen
- To restore metabolism, we must consume the amount of water our body needs.
- Water provides the oxygen the body needs to produce energy and keep our metabolism in motion.
- Drinking the right amount of water produces the following benefits, among many others:
  - restores metabolism
    - increases energy levels
    - removes acids and toxins from the body
    - helps slim down

- lowers blood pressure
- helps with constipation and good digestion
- helps control diabetes
- improves sexual performance
- improves the overall health of the body

Answer the following questions

1. Determine the correct number of glasses of water per day that your body needs.

    Your weight is _____ (pounds / kilograms). Divide your total weight by 16, if in pounds, or by 7 if in kilograms. Write the number resulting from the division here _____.

    So, you should consume daily _____ glasses of water (8 oz or 250 ml). _(weight divided by 16 or 7)

2. Why is it vitally important that you consume at least this amount of water per day?

3. What decision have you made and what actions will you take after understanding the importance of staying hydrated?

WE ARE ALL DIFFERENT

At this point I must explain one of the most important discoveries that has made metabolic technology [64] so successful, both in reducing body fat (slimming down) and in controlling diabetes. Notice that the problem with diets, all of them (calorie reduction, fat reduction, eating less, etc.), is that people generally manage to lose weight, but soon after they suffer from the famous "weight rebound", which makes them put on weight again, often more than the initial weight at which they had started dieting.

Diets do not really work unless you improve your metabolism. More than twenty years and hundreds of thousands of people served at NaturalSlim allowed us to realize that the failure of diets to slim down or to control diabetes had to do with a person's lack of knowledge of how their metabolism works. Those who are suffering and failing from one diet to the next, all have a slow metabolism.

Just as there are a handful of people who can eat whatever they want and never get fat, it is also true that most of us get fat too easily, due to the phenomenon of slow metabolism. For those of us who suffer from a slow metabolism, it seems that we get fat even by looking at

---

[64] technology: is the name given to a collection of knowledge that is applied in an orderly manner to achieve desired results or effects. A real technology can always produce predictable results.

food. However, we all know at least one of those very thin people (I affectionately call them "those damn skinny people") who can eat pizza, fatty foods, chocolate, sweets and sugary sodas all day long and simply do not put on weight, no matter what they eat. A slow metabolism is nothing more than an inefficient metabolism. Since the body's metabolism is what creates the body's energy, any problem of inefficiency in your metabolism will be reflected in a deficiency of energy production.

The first thing we must understand is that metabolism creates the body's energy. It is the energy of the body that enables movement. Nothing can move unless there is first an energy to move it. All the body's processes depend on achieving an appropriate level of energy creation from the metabolism. It is also necessary that the amount of energy created, and its speed of movement is at the appropriate rhythm, not too fast, not too slow.

My observation is that the human body is an organism of exquisite design and great precision, which does not tolerate excesses of anything, neither too hot, nor too cold, nor too acidic, nor too alkaline (opposite of acid), nor too much food, nor too much hunger, and so on. The human body tries at all costs to maintain internal METABOLIC BALANCE, which is called homeostasis[65]. The

---

[65] homeostasis: is a compound word from the Greek *homo* meaning similar and *stasis* meaning state or stability. Homeostasis is a property of living organisms that consists of their ability to maintain a stable internal condition, using metabolism to compensate for changes in their environment (food, temperature, hydration, etc.). It is a form of dynamic equilibrium, made possible by a network of control systems in the human body.

subject of METABOLIC BALANCE is so important to the body that you do not even have to think about maintaining it; your body does it automatically using the AUTONOMOUS Nervous System[66].

To understand how the nervous system works, first we must understand which are the parts that compose it. Let's start by saying that the brain, which is the command center, is part of the nervous system and from there all the functions of the body are directed.

The nervous system is a communication system made up of the brain and nerves, with an extensive wiring system that transmits electrical impulses produced by the brain to order all other systems in the body to function.

For your heart to pump blood, the nervous system sends out electrical impulses that tell the heart to contract. Likewise, the nervous system sends electrical impulses that cause your lungs to inhale and exhale air for breathing. There are also electrical impulses that direct what happens in your stomach for digestion, and electrical impulses so that your intestine moves and your leg muscles coordinate so that you can walk.

---

[66] AUTONOMOUS Nervous System: is the part of the nervous system that controls the body's involuntary actions (that you do not have to think about). The AUTONOMOUS Nervous System controls the heart, lungs, pancreas, liver, intestine, and all the body's vital hormonal processes. It is what causes the heart rate to accelerate automatically when someone is frightened, for blood pressure to rise, or blood glucose to rise in a diabetic, even if he or she has not eaten. It is called AUTONOMOUS because it cannot be controlled by the mind; it operates independently of a person's thoughts.

In short, all the movements your body needs to perform to maintain life are controlled by the electrical impulses that your brain emits and that are transmitted through your nervous system. Let's see how the nervous system is structured.

Note that the nervous system is divided into two parts: the first is what we call the CENTRAL Nervous System, which is composed of the brain and the spinal cord [67], through which all the nerves that carry the electrical impulses that originate in the brain pass.

The second part of the nervous system is called the PERIPHERAL [68] Nervous System. It is called peripheral because it comprises nerves that are in the periphery, that is, on the sides or around the spinal cord. The PERIPHERAL Nervous System receives the electrical impulses from the spinal cord to be distributed to all the other multiple systems of the body.

---

[67] spinal medulla: this is that large bundle of different nerves that travel from the brain through the entire length of the spinal cord and carry the electrical impulses that control all the movements of the body.

[68] peripheral: this is the name given to one of the subdivisions of the nervous system. It comes from the word periphery, which refers to the area immediately outside a space.

The Nervous System is initially divided into:

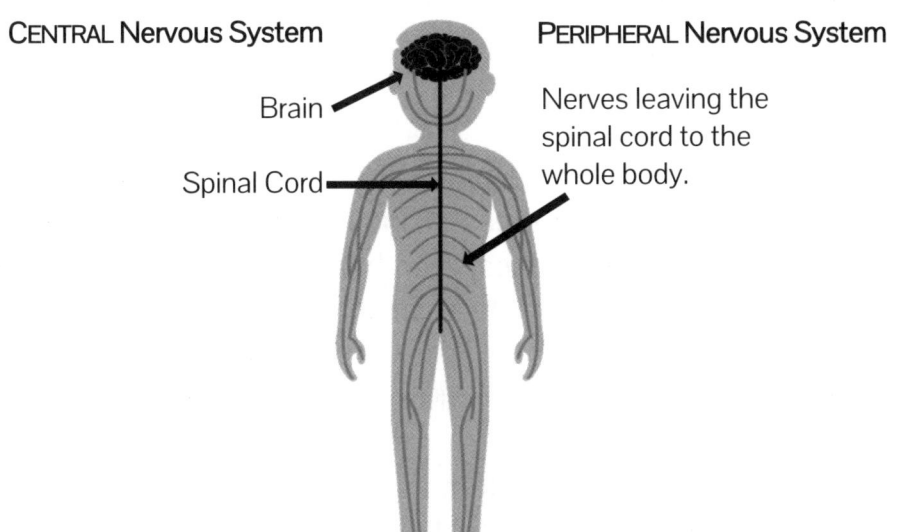

To summarize, these first two major divisions of the nervous system are divided between the CENTRAL Nervous System, which comprises the brain, from where the electrical nerve impulses originate, and the spinal cord which will distribute those electrical nerve impulses to the second part, which is the PERIPHERAL Nervous System.

So, when we talk about the heart pumping blood, this happens because the electrical nerve impulse that starts in the brain goes down the spinal cord, which is the first part, and from there it goes to the second part, which is the PERIPHERAL Nervous System that carries those impulses to make the heart work.

In the same way, when the impulses go from the spinal cord to the lungs, breathing is achieved. Likewise, when they go to the stomach, digestion is achieved. When the electrical impulses go to the intestine, intestinal movement is achieved and when they go to the leg muscles, walking is achieved.

The PERIPHERAL Nervous System is the one that allows the nerve impulses coming from the brain to reach organs such as the lungs, liver, heart and also connects with glands such as the thyroid, pancreas or adrenal glands. So, the peripheral system extends the domain of the brain's control over all other parts of the body.

The PERIPHERAL System has a part that functions in an involuntary manner which is called the AUTONOMOUS Nervous System. It is called AUTONOMOUS because it functions in an automatic or independent manner and cannot be controlled at will. It is an independent and automatic system that controls or influences all the other systems of the body.

The AUTONOMOUS System controls your breathing, heartbeat, digesting your food, and even generate sweat to lower your body temperature. You can consciously control some of these automatic actions such as breathing deeply or slowing down, but you do not have to command your body to breathe as this is an involuntary action carried out by your AUTONOMOUS System to ensure that you do not die from lack of oxygen.

The body's AUTONOMOUS Nervous System runs on automatic, twenty-four hours a day, every day of your life, trying to maintain a METABOLIC BALANCE. Achieving that state of METABOLIC BALANCE is so important to the body that it will naturally do what it can to slow down any internal processes that are happening too quickly. It will also try to speed up any process that is too slow.

In short, your body continuously and permanently struggles to maintain the metabolic equilibrium or balance because it depends on achieving internal movements and changes at an optimal rate (not too fast, not too slow) to survive.

Any situation that is extreme puts the body at risk. For this reason, having constipation (a bowel movement that is too slow) can be just as problematic as having the opposite which would be diarrhea (a bowel movement that is too fast). Having a fast heart rate, heart palpitations[69], is just as dangerous as having one that is too slow. Having a temperature that is too high, which we call fever, and which is produced by an excess of activity and movements of the immune system in its fight against bacteria, can be just as dangerous as having a temperature that is too low (hypothermia[70]). The human body depends on its METABOLIC BALANCE for health.

---

[69] cardiac palpitations: if your heart rate is too fast (more than 100 beats per minute), it is called tachycardia, if it is too slow it is called bradycardia, and if it is irregular, it is called arrhythmia. Any abnormal rhythm condition is cause for concern.

[70] hypothermia: means that the body temperature is too low, as would be experienced by someone suffering from the crushing cold of the North Pole, from which they may die. It also happens to shipwrecked survivors who are forced to float for a long time at sea where the water temperature is too cold.

When it comes to metabolism, it is crucial that the internal processes of the body's cells occur at an appropriate speed, which is neither too fast nor too slow. The nervous system controls the nerve impulses which, in turn, control the speed of metabolic processes.

In the same way that your heart needs to maintain a rate of palpitations within a normal range to be healthy, the cells of the body, which is where the creation of the energy that produces metabolism occurs, must also maintain an adequate speed in their internal chemical processes. For this, the body must always manage to maintain a regulation of the acidity or alkalinity[71] (opposite of acidity) of the cells. To restore the metabolism, it is first necessary to understand it and then take the correct actions to restore METABOLIC BALANCE.

We already know that all vital body processes such as breathing, digestion, elimination, defenses, circulation and other systems are controlled by the brain, through the AUTONOMOUS Nervous System, through electrical impulses that travel through the nerves of the nervous system, which would be the equivalent of the electrical wiring in your house.

The AUTONOMOUS System, in turn, is divided into two parts called the SYMPATHETIC Nervous System[72] and the

---

[71] acidity or alkalinity: it is measured on the "pH" scale, which stands for "potential of hydrogen". The more hydrogen a substance contains, the more acidic it is, the less hydrogen it contains, the more alkaline it is. You can see the pH scale in the glossary section of this book.

[72] SYMPATHETIC Nervous System: that part of the nervous system that reacts to stress and threats by raising blood pressure, increasing heart rate, and preparing the body to fight or run.

PARASYMPATHETIC Nervous System[73]. However, for the sake of keeping the language simple, I decided to rename them as the EXCITED[74] Nervous System and the PASSIVE Nervous System. I named them this way to avoid technical words that do not really facilitate the understanding of people who do not have an education in medicine:

The Two Divisions of the AUTONOMOUS Nervous System			
Physicians call it	Its function is to	It is equivalent to	We rename it as
Sympathetic Nervous System	create or accelerate movements	the ACCELERATOR pedal of your car	EXCITED Nervous System
Parasympathetic Nervous System	stop or decelerate movements	the BRAKE pedal of your car	PASSIVE Nervous System

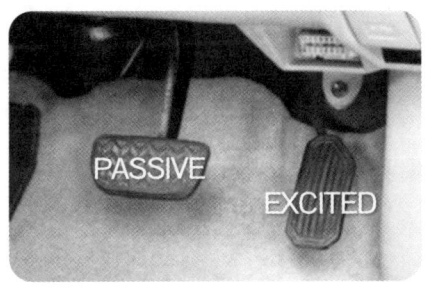

---

[73] PARASYMPATHETIC Nervous System: that part of the nervous system that slows the heart rate and relaxes the musculature to allow rest and relaxation, or deep, restorative sleep.
[74] excited: this name proved to be very effective so that the people that we were helping with the metabolism could learn it, associate it, and remember it, although I had to clarify to my friends from Mexico that "excited" has nothing to do with sexuality, since in their country "excited" has a sexual connotation.

I always try to choose the simplest language I can to explain our metabolism technology, always seeking the understanding of the person I want to help. I make an enormous effort to keep the words and examples I use simple, because I know that the results obtained by the person will depend solely on his or her understanding of these subjects. For this reason, from here on out, I will refer to these two parts of the AUTONOMOUS Nervous System simply as **EXCITED** and **PASSIVE**.

Although since 2006 when my book *The Power of Your Metabolism* was published, I have been able to help thousands of people throughout Latin America and the world, I always keep researching with the goal of helping people even more. So, after four years of research, I discovered that **the AUTONOMOUS Nervous System plays a crucial role in metabolism**. I discovered that the sequence of metabolic control is as follows:

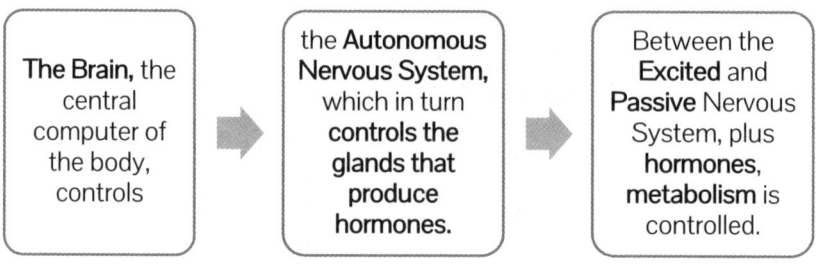

More importantly, I discovered, thanks to the work of other researchers who were pioneers in the fields of nutrition and physiology[75], that the different foods in the

---

[75] physiology: physiology, from the Greek *physis* "nature" and *logos* "knowledge or study". It is the biological science that studies the functioning of living beings.

diet had their own effects of either exciting or calming the nervous system. For example, red meat and fat excite the nervous system, while vegetables and salad have a calming effect. The same goes for vitamins and minerals; for example, calcium excites, and magnesium and potassium calm and relax the nervous system.

In fact, I discovered that I could improve anyone's metabolism if I chose the right foods to recommended for their diet. That opened my eyes to new possibilities for managing obesity and hormone imbalance conditions such as diabetes.

However, the most important of all, was the discovery that WE ARE ALL DIFFERENT therefore, diets cannot be the same for everyone. I discovered that some of us have more active or more dominant Excited Nervous System and others, have more active or dominant, Passive Nervous System.

This discovery, when applied to our metabolism consulting practice at the NaturalSlim centers, greatly improved the results we obtained. Invariably, when we apply it, we make people slim down faster, with less effort, with a higher energy level and even with a better quality of sleep.

The Two Sides Of The Nervous System: Excited and Passive

The part of the nervous system that we call the EXCITED side activates the glands and organs that defend the body from an attack. The attack may be real (someone threatening you with a gun, bacteria attacking the body), or imagined, like saying you are afraid of being fired from your job. Regardless of how a threat is perceived, your nervous system will react by activating the aroused side of the nervous system to defend itself.

The EXCITED system handles threats, so it prepares the body to fight or flee. The nerves of the Excited Nervous System make more blood and nutrients go to the brain and muscles to help fight the threat. The EXCITED system also stimulates and activates the thyroid and adrenal glands to provide a greater amount of energy in order to fight or flee from danger.

When the Excited Nervous System is activated, the heart rhythm and blood pressure increase, while the blood flow to the digestive and elimination system is reduced. Note that when someone gets scared or is having a bad time, the heartbeat rhythm increases, and the person's blood pressure (tension) rises. Also, when the Excited Nervous System reacts as if there is a threat, glucose rises, even if you have not eaten in five to six hours, because to combat the perceived threat, your body will release glucose that is stored in the liver, in the form of glycogen[76]. Any situation in which you are feeling nervous, stressed, or having feelings of panic is the result of an Excited Nervous System that has been activated.

An overactive Excited Nervous System, when maintained with excessive activity, is destructive for the body. You can observe how a person ages and looks emaciated when he or she has lost a loved one or has been going through an overly stressful situation. Accelerated physical deterioration is the result of an EXCITED system that is kept in a constant state of alertness. When there is an alert situation and the EXCITED system is activated, all the body's energy is reserved for the defense, so no energy is left to nourish the cells or to eliminate toxics. People become stressed and get constipation because the EXCITED system stops the bowel movement and reserves all its resources for a fight-or-flight response. When the EXCITED system is on a state of alert for too long, it is like a country putting its entire army on alert to prepare for war. While the whole country is on alert, with its army ready to defend the country, the economic activity of that country will suffer serious damage, and the country will become poorer every day. Something similar happens to the body. If the EXCITED system remains in a state of alert for an extended period, a person's health will begin to decline, starting with their quality of sleep, which will become very poor.

---

[76] glycogen: a type of starch (imagine mashed potatoes) that the liver creates naturally to store glucose. This allows it to keep blood glucose levels stable between meals. Glycogen is like a combustible reserve that is stored in the liver and muscles until the body needs it to increase blood glucose levels.

On the other hand, the PASSIVE side of the nervous system has its nerves connected to everything that has to do with nourishing, healing, or regenerating the body. The PASSIVE side is a system that builds or repairs parts of the body, while the EXCITED system destroys parts of the body. The nerves of the PASSIVE system stimulate digestion, the immune system and the elimination organs. These organs that are under the control of the PASSIVE system include the liver, the pancreas, the stomach, and the intestines.

When a threat exists and the EXCITED system is activated, the PASSIVE system is deactivated, which may damage your digestion, make you sick because the immune system is reduced, or cause you to suffer from elimination problems, such as constipation, while you are under the effects of stressful situations. To regain health and restore metabolism it is necessary for the body to spend a greater amount of time not suffering from the wear and tear that an Excited Nervous System causes.

The Excited Nervous System and the Passive Nervous System are the opposite of each other. One or the other is always activated, but never at the same time. In the car, you either step on the gas or put on the brakes, but not at the same time. The EXCITED system takes prominence over the PASSIVE.

To heal the body, you must achieve METABOLIC BALANCE and that is achieved, among other recommendations in this book, by choosing foods correctly for your dominant type of nervous system, which can be either EXCITED or PASSIVE. All extremes are bad, so an overly Excited Nervous System is just as bad as an overly PASSIVE one. Life and health must be kept in balance.

How To Identify Your Type of Nervous System

First, you must understand that you are a spiritual being, and you are NOT your body. Beings have ideas, opinions, attitudes, preferences, and aspirations because we are SPIRITUAL BEINGS. You are not your body, just as you are not your car. You, as a being, are the owner of your body and make the necessary decisions to take care or neglect your body. Your body does not make decisions, it has no opinions, no political preferences, nor any aspirations.

Your body is your body, period. It is an organism that possesses life and senses that allow you to enjoy the game of life. I explain this because when it comes to determining whether your BODY has an Excited or Passive Nervous System, what we are evaluating is THE BODY, not YOU who is the SPIRITUAL BEING.

Among the members of the NaturalSlim System, I frequently meet someone who is confused about this issue of EXCITED or PASSIVE and says: "one of your consultants told me that I am PASSIVE, but I feel that I am excited, because I am always in a hurry, I am impatient, and it bothers me to wait". In a case like this, the person is confusing his or her body with him or herself, which is the person. What has an Excited Nervous System or Passive Nervous System is the body, not the person. Your body has diabetes or a slow metabolism, not you.

The subject is confusing because there are people who have a great deal of serenity and are very calm as people, while they have an Excited Nervous System body that suffers from insomnia, poor sleep, poor digestion and constipation, as it happens to those with an Excited Nervous System. If you observe someone who is very calm you might mistakenly think, "they must be PASSIVE", something that is not necessarily true. There are also people whose body has a Passive Nervous System, while they, as beings, are extremely active, cannot sit still for a minute, are irritable and behave in a certain state of excitement. Do not get confused between you and your body. The Excited or Passive Nervous System has to do only with your body.

To determine whether your nervous system is EXCITED or PASSIVE, you only need to answer a simple test. The test consists of five indicators. These are the five most common manifestations that bodies with an Excited Nervous System have.

These five indicators reflect five characteristics of the EXCITED, which we have discovered in the metabolism research, that best reflect the type of nervous system that is dominant in your body.

The rule is this:

If you answer YES to any of these five questions, <u>even if it is only one of them and even if it is with "only once in a while"</u>, you have a body whose nervous system is EXCITED.

Those of us with a Passive Nervous System always answer **NO** to each of the following five indicators:

	Excited Nervous System Indicators
1	I have trouble digesting red meat or it takes time to digest it (if you do not eat red meat, consider what would happen if you did)
2	Consuming saturated fat or fatty foods, such as pork, pork chops or fried foods, can cause me digestive problems
3	If I eat late at night, I don't digest well
4	Consuming food after a certain time at night, can make it difficult for me to sleep (I am slow to fall asleep)
5	I am a light sleeper and extreme noises, or movements can easily wake me up (shallow sleep)

To how many of the indicators did you answer **YES**? If you answered that you suffer from one or more of these five indicators, you should consider that your body has an Excited Nervous System. If you did not check any of the five indicators, your body has a Passive Nervous System. We will see later on what the recommendations of the types of foods would be that it would be convenient for you to consume as part of your 3x1 Diet, in order to obtain the best results in the control of your diabetes and in achieving slimming down, if that is something you are missing.

At this point you should know whether your body has a nervous system that is predominantly EXCITED or PASSIVE. If you are in doubt or think "I have a little bit of both, EXCITED and PASSIVE ", there was simply something you did not understand in the above explanation. All our bodies have both the Excited and Passive Nervous Systems because both parts of the nervous system are necessary to sustain life. What we are trying to assess to help you improve the efficiency of your metabolism is, which of the two parts of the AUTONOMOUS Nervous System (EXCITED or PASSIVE) is more dominant in your body?

These two parts of the AUTONOMOUS Nervous System (EXCITED and PASSIVE) are equally important, just like the gas pedal and brake pedal in your car. Your body has both. What happens is that, from a metabolism perspective, we have discovered that we all have, mainly because of hereditary factors, a certain more pronounced inclination towards one of the two sides: more EXCITED or more PASSIVE. There are some bodies that have the "gas pedal" (EXCITED) activated most of the time, while there are other bodies that stay longer with the "brake pedal" (PASSIVE) activated.

When we try to detect whether your body's nervous system is predominantly EXCITED or whether it is PASSIVE, what we are trying to do is to better understand what is going on with your metabolism, and with your body's capacity for energy creation. Both the Excited Nervous System that is overly EXCITED, and the Passive Nervous System that is overly PASSIVE, are out of balance. This is reflected in a person's lack of energy, who is exhausted, with poor sleep quality, with constipation, with a lazy thyroid (hypothyroidism) or too accelerated (hyperthyroidism) and, in diabetics, with an out of control of glucose, simply because the metabolism is being thrown out of control by the wrong diet for his type of system.

In principle, we are looking for a balance using the properties of the foods of the 3x1 Diet that we are going to use to calm the body, reducing what would be an excess of stimulation with red meat and fat, to those who have an Excited Nervous System. We also seek to balance, with a higher consumption of foods that are exciting to the nervous system (red meat, crustaceans such as shrimp or lobster, fatty fish such as salmon or tuna, fatty cheeses), to stimulate a nervous system that is too PASSIVE.

Theoretically, there must be someone who has a perfect balance between his EXCITED and PASSIVE system, but for sure, he neither suffers from diabetes nor obesity; both diabetes and obesity are caused by a metabolic imbalance, which then affects the hormonal system and becomes the out-of-control glucose of a diabetic, or in the excess of glucose that produces the excessive fat that we call obesity.

If you are still not sure as to whether your body has a predominantly Excited or Passive Nervous System, read the previous section again and make sure to clarify with a dictionary any word you find that does not help the material make sense to you. Lack of comprehension of any subject only comes from not understanding the meaning of the words being used. Remember that there are words that have different meanings, depending on how they are used.

An additional thing you can do to clarify the topic is to visit MetabolismoTV and do a search under EXCITED or PASSIVE. You will find about 20+ short videos that explain the topic of EXCITED or PASSIVE in greater detail. There is a video titled "Dominant Characteristics of the Excited" (Episode #199). By watching that video, you will find answers to your questions. The better you master this topic and know whether your body has a predominantly Excited or Passive Nervous System the easier it will be to restore your metabolism.

Pathway to an Ultra-Powerful Metabolism

👀 **To restore our metabolism we must correctly identify which Type of Nervous System is predominant in our body.**
- The AUTONOMOUS Nervous System is composed of an extensive wiring of nerves that run from our brain and spinal cord throughout the body. The AUTONOMOUS Nervous System controls the involuntary actions of the body. It controls the heart, the lungs, the pancreas, the liver, the intestine and all the body's vital hormonal processes.
- The AUTONOMOUS Nervous System is divided into two types of systems with different functions that guarantee our survival. The two types of nervous systems are the EXCITED and the PASSIVE.
- The Excited Nervous System manages the threats, so it prepares the body to fight or flight. The nerves of the Excited Nervous System get more blood and nutrients to the brain and to the muscles to help fight the threat. When it is activated for too long, it has devastating effects on the body.

👀 **Answer the following questions**
1. Identify which type of nervous system is predominant in your body by checking all the conditions that apply to you from the following list:

_____ I have trouble digesting red meat or it takes time to digest it (if you do not eat red meat, consider what would happen if you did).

_____ Consuming saturated fat or fatty foods, such as pork, pork chops or fried foods, can cause me digestive problems.

_____ If I eat late at night, I don't digest well.

_____ Consuming food after a certain time at night can make it difficult for me to sleep (I take a long time to fall asleep).

_____ I am a light sleeper and extreme noises, or movements can easily wake me up (shallow sleep).

How many of the indicators did you check?
_____

If you checked at least one of these five indicators, your nervous system is EXCITED. Excited Nervous System people have one or more of the five conditions. True PASSIVES answer NO to all of them.

2. According to the selected indicators, write here your type of nervous system.

3. What decision have you made and what actions will you take, after having identified your type of nervous system?

THE 3x1 DIET
TO RESTORE METABOLISM

In reality, the 3x1 Diet, more than a diet, is a LIFESTYLE. The word diet always makes us think of prohibitions or starving ourselves by counting calories. However, the word diet comes from the Greek *dayta*, which means "regime of life".

The 3x1 Diet is a FORM OF COMBINING FOODS that allows you to eat whatever you like and still slim down or control diabetes. In the 3x1 Diet there are no forbidden foods; all types of foods are allowed. The important thing is to maintain the correct PROPORTION between what we call **Type S Foods** (SLIMMING – SUPPORT the control of diabetes) and **Type F Foods** (FATTENING – act as a FOE (ENEMIES) to the control of diabetes). Look at the following table explaining that **Type S Foods** help us slim down and control diabetes because they are foods that don't produce a large amount of glucose (blood sugar). You will see that, on the contrary, **Type F Foods** produce a large amount of glucose, so they will make a diabetic put on weight or raise their glucose.

It is very important that we clearly understand the difference between the foods that harm us and the foods that help us to improve our metabolism. I call **Type F Foods** that way because they are the foods that make us **Fat** and they are also the **Foe** foods of diabetes control and they are basically the refined carbohydrates and the rest of the foods that produce way to much glucose in the body, preventing us from being able to slim down. Let us see what foods make up this group in more detail.

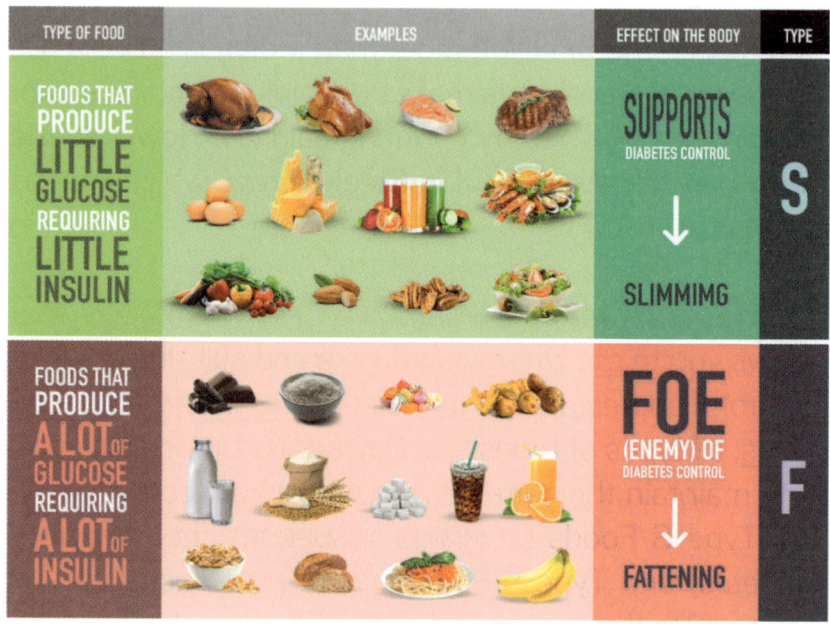

EXPANDED LIST OF TYPE F FOODS – FATTENING

cereals
rice, oatmeal, corn flour, farina, cornstarch, corn flakes, bran flakes, corn pops, muesli, pancakes, mini wheats, frosted flakes, etc.

breads
white bread, sweet bread, "sobao bread", water bread, butter bread, hot dog bread, hamburger bread, ciabatta, bagels, croissants,

biscuits, sweet cookies, soda crackers, wafers, croissants, soy flours, pita, potato bread, salted crackers, pizza, bruschetta, corn bread, whole wheat bread

pastas
ALL (noodles, spaghetti, etc.)

other farinaceous
white and brown rice, potatoes, beans, chickpeas, pigeon peas,

corn, sweet peas, sweet potato, yucca, yams, "yautia", squash, green bananas, "malanga", plantains, jasmine rice, tortillas for tacos and burrito.

vegetables
cooked onion, tomato, cooked carrot, beet, corn

milk
fresh, UHT, evaporated, condensed, lactose-free, Lactaid milk

sweeteners
sugar, honey, corn syrup, glucose, sucrose, fructose, lactose, agave syrup, brown sugar, turbinado sugar, maltose, molasses, maple syrup

fruits
dried plums, raisins, watermelon, figs, pineapple, all fruits packed in syrup, papaya, guava, banana, melons, honey dew, cantaloupe, mangos, kiwi, dates, grapes, oranges, grapefruit, peach, apricot, plums

beverages
carbonated soft drinks (ALL), fruit nectars, pineapple, grape, cranberry, plum, orange juices; milk shakes, alcoholic beverages, fruit drinks (juice drinks), chocolate drinks, commercial carrot juice

condiments
sugar toppings, ketchup, BBQ sauce, jellies, jams, marmalades, peanut butter, syrup, pancake syrup

Now, this may sound alarming and restrictive, but it is not. The trick is to know the proportion in which these fattening foods will be combined with the slimming ones. As I like to give you good news, here I include in detail what are those foods that help us.

Expanded List of Type S Foods – Slimming

poultry
chicken, turkey, and quail

fish
mahi mahi, grouper, snapper, salmon, tilapia, cod, turbot, skipper, mackerel, hake, tuna

seafood
crab meat, shrimp, crab, octopus, squid, oysters, oysters, mackerel, lobster, scallops, mussels, clams

cheeses
country white, cheddar, American, Swiss, gouda, edam, parmesan, ricotta, mozzarella, Monterrey, provolone, muenster, camembert, stilton, cream cheese, brie, Manchego

milk
almond milk (no sugar added), heavy cream, half and half, coconut milk

beef
ground beef, steak, skirt steak, chuck, tenderloin, filet, suckling pig, liver, steaks, sirloin, tenderloin

pork meat
chops, ribs, pork leg, pork loin, bacon,

vegetables
olives, avocado, celery, broccoli, chayote, brussels sprouts, cabbage, green beans, spinach, asparagus, lettuce (all), peppers (all), mushrooms, raw carrots, pickles, cauliflower, raw onions, tomatoes

fruits
strawberries, apples

condiments
basil, garlic, mustard, paprika, oregano, recao, coriander, sage, mint, rosemary, pepper, bay leaves, Worcestershire sauce, soy sauce, vinegar

fats
olive oil, coconut oil, linseed oil, avocado, almond, sesame, grapeseed, butter

nuts
almonds, hazelnuts, peanuts, pecans, walnuts, macadamias, pistachios, and sunflower and pumpkin seeds

sweeteners
low carb natural sweetener, stevia, maltitol

As we have already seen, for the body to create new fat and gain weight, glucose and insulin must always be combined. Insulin is the hormone that allows the body's cells to utilize glucose. When you combine a lot of glucose with a lot of insulin you will always get more new fat creation. Let's review how the body creates new fat and you become fat:

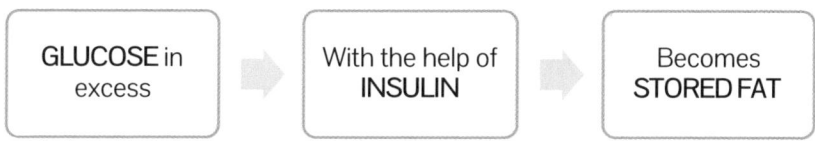

You should know that in this process of fat creation you have a hormone that is your ally. In the same way that the insulin hormone is a storage hormone (insulin stores fat, builds and grows muscles and tissues), there is another hormone that is also produced by the pancreas that has an opposite effect to insulin. The hormone that has the opposite of insulin's effect is called glucagon and we could say that it is a repartitioning hormone. For example, insulin stores fat and glucagon remove fat from the body. Insulin reduces blood glucose (to feed the cells or to convert glucose into fat) and glucagon increases blood glucose so that the cells have their support.

When you reduce your intake of refined carbohydrates and starches the glucose in your blood is also naturally reduced. If the reduction in glucose is significant enough, the body will react by increasing its production of glucagon[77] to increase the availability of glucose in the blood. This is precisely the mechanism that makes someone who is overweight slim down because by reducing the consumption of Type F Foods, glucose is reduced, the body reacts by producing a greater amount of glucagon and glucagon extracts the stored glucose from the liver in order to bring glucose levels to a normal level. In addition, glucagon signals the body to use its fat reserves to feed the cells and you begin to slim down.

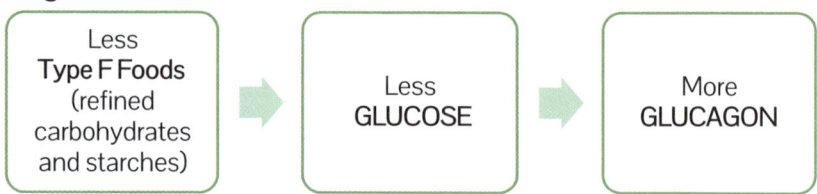

To slim down and restore metabolism, there needs to be a balance between insulin production (converts excess glucose into fat) and glucagon production (breaks down stored fat). That is why it is important that you eat only your three meals and avoid snacking. If you eat breakfast and two hours later have a snack, you are forcing the pancreas to produce more insulin hormone again to pick up the glucose from the food you just ate and get it into the cells. However, if you do not eat anything between meals, you are allowing blood glucose levels to drop and forcing the pancreas to produce the hormone glucagon. Among other things, the glucagon hormone will break down the fat you have stored to

---

[77] glucagon: a hormone produced by the pancreas that has the effect of reducing hunger and helps burn stored body fat (obesity), thus having the opposite effect of insulin, which is a hormone that causes hunger and accumulates fat.

convert it into glucose and feed the cells, which will definitely make you slim down.

So, we could say that, for those who wish to slim down, glucagon is a friend because it helps to mobilize the body's fat, and excessive insulin is their enemy because it makes them fat. In fact, if there is a high level of insulin in the body, the use of stored body fat is totally inhibited. So, by making only your three meals, in the proper combination of Type S Foods and Type F Foods you are guaranteed to lose fat from your body. The correct way to combine these foods is the 3x1 Diet.

The 3x1 Diet teaches you how to proportion your plate so that you do not create an excess of glucose, that way you will be able to slim down, control diabetes and improve your body's metabolism. Damage to the body always occurs when glucose rises too high, so by controlling the portion of Type F Foods you eat, you will be avoiding damage to your health. The obesity and diabetes epidemic affecting the population is caused by an excess of Type F Foods. When you learn to use the proportions of the 3x1 Diet you will be controlling your body's hormonal system and you will feel that your body's energy has increased.

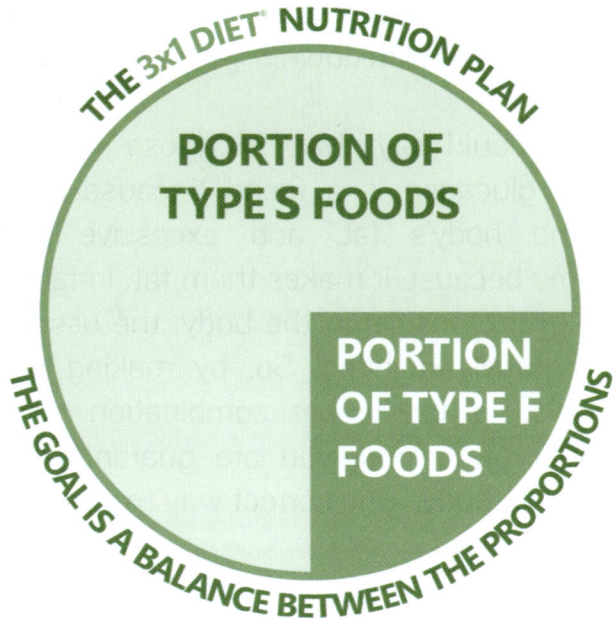

The 3x1 Diet can be used in a restaurant, cafeteria or at home, as it only depends on whether you know how to classify foods as Type S or Type F, which is very easy to do. Type S Foods, which are those that make you SLIM and those that helps SUPPORT the control of diabetes, should always occupy ¾ of your plate. Type F Foods, which are those that make you FAT and act as a FOE (ENEMIES) for the control of diabetes, should only occupy ¼ portion of your plate. By doing this, you will be achieving a proportion between Type S and Type F that will keep glucose (blood sugar) levels at a healthy level. See below different examples of the 3x1 Diet and how a dish of food is proportioned between Type S Foods and Type F Foods:

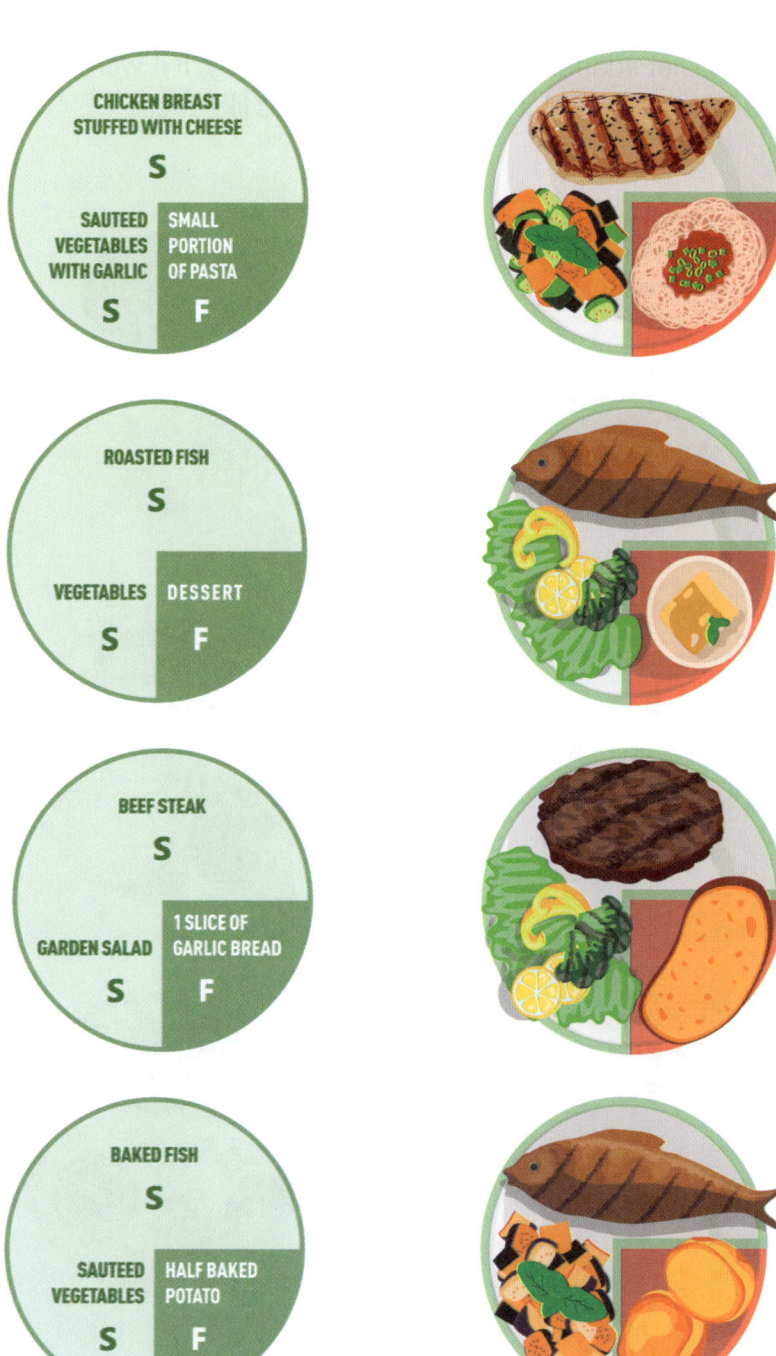

The 3x1 Diet adapts to the food of any country. If it were to be used "Mexican style" it would be examples like these:

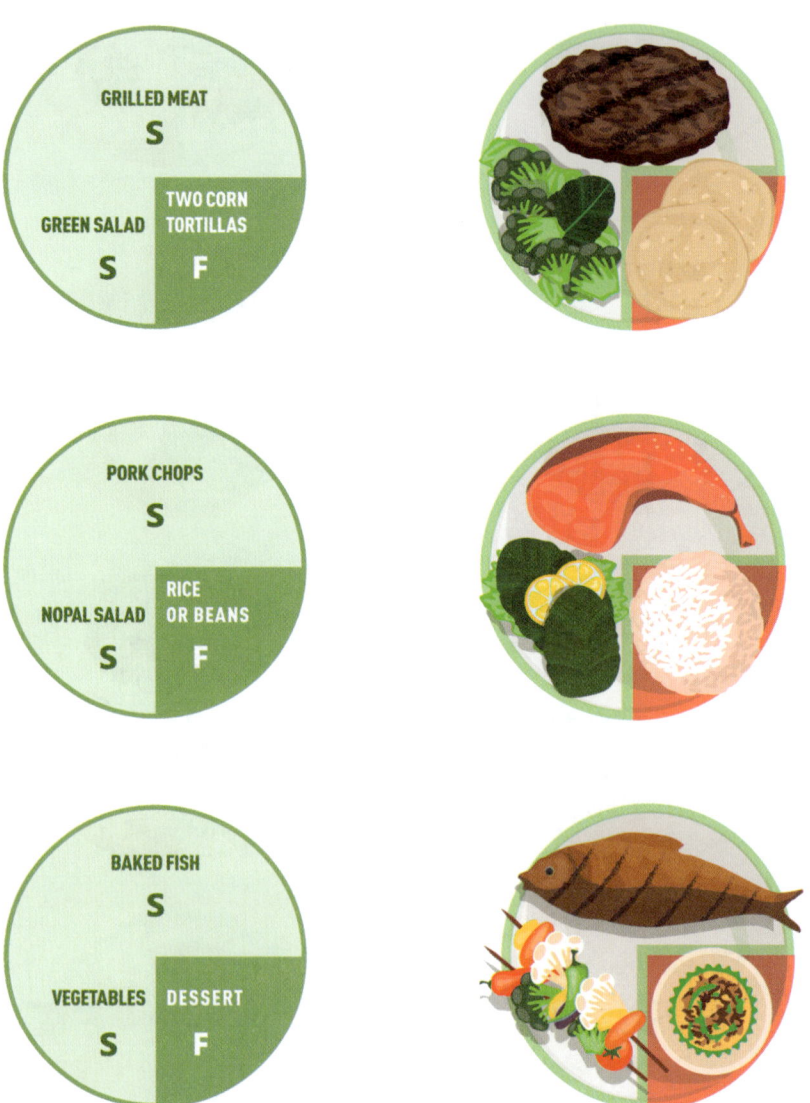

The 3x1 Diet also applies to breakfasts from all countries:

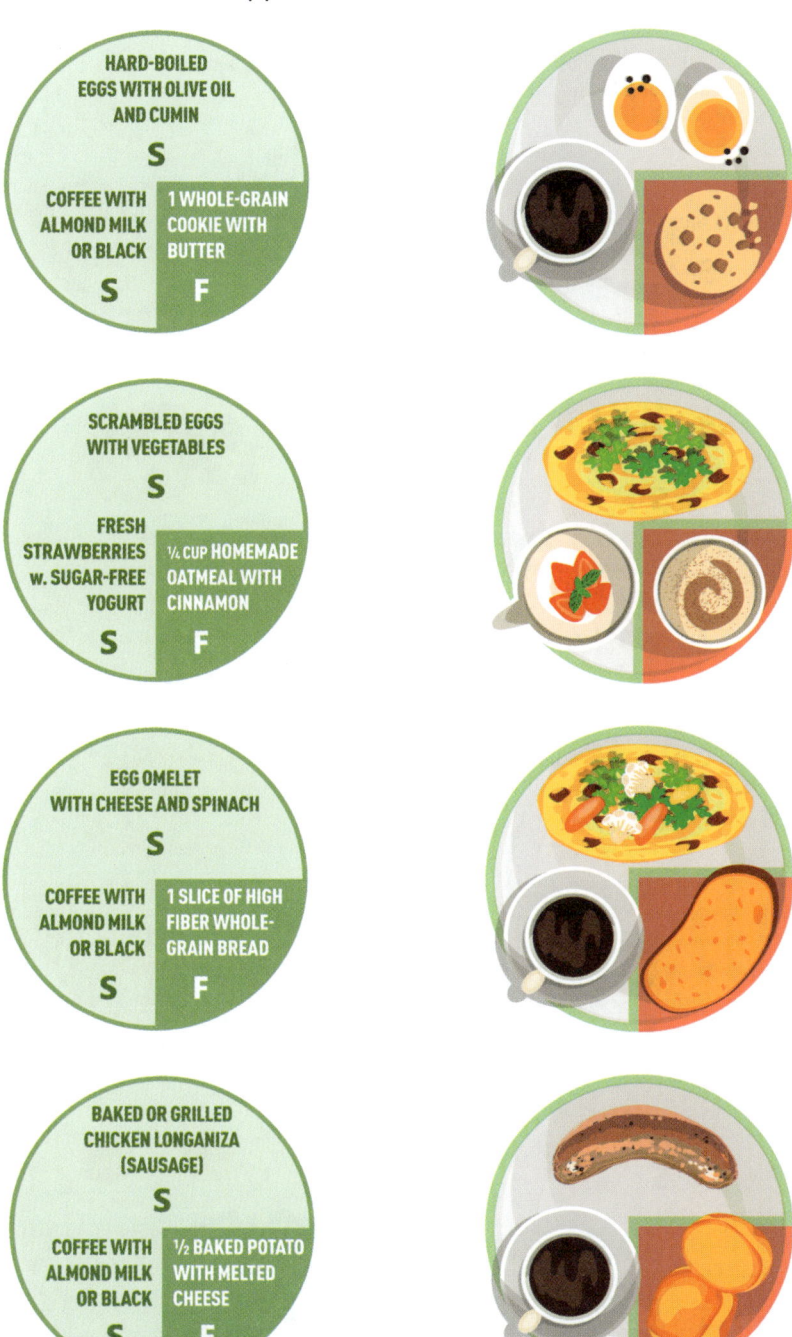

For example, breakfast in Mexico could be combined like this:

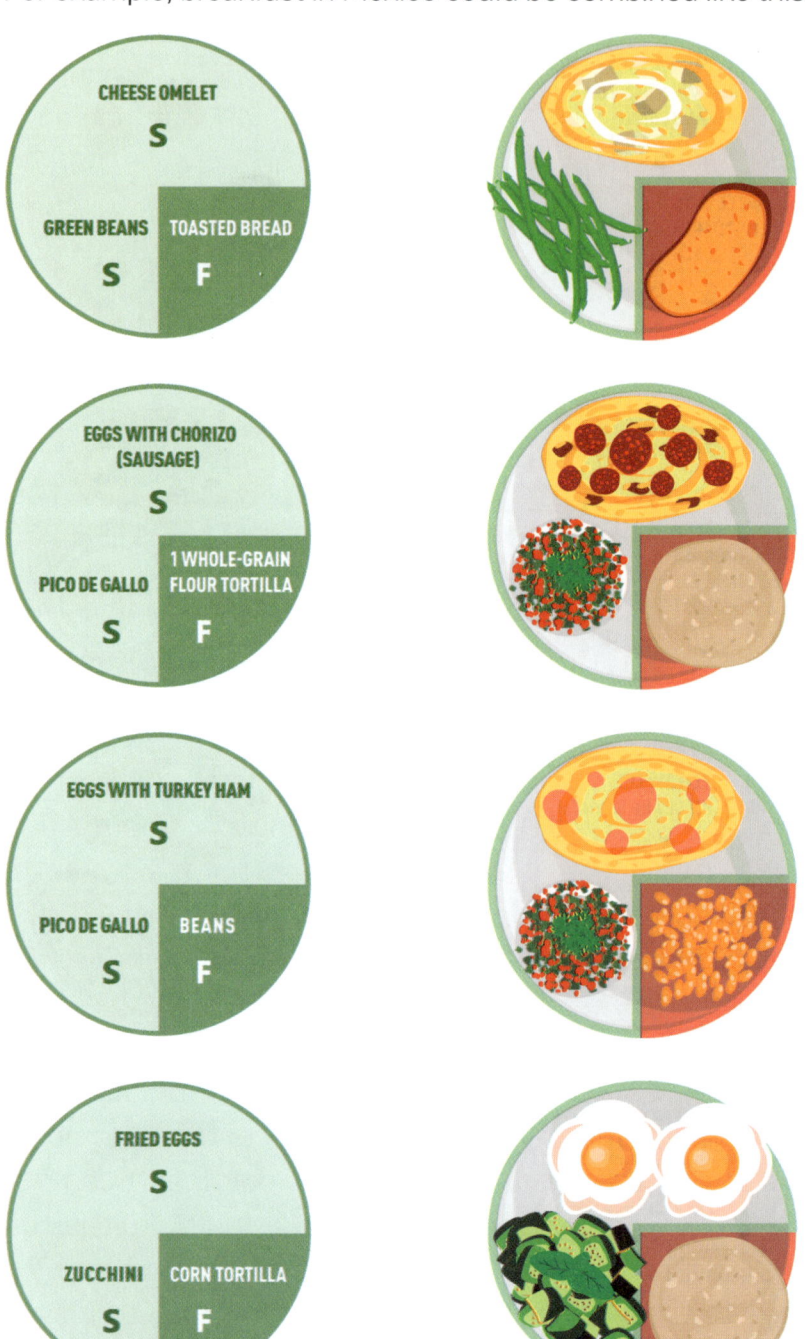

The basic concept of proportions between Type S and Type F Foods is also applicable to soups or broths. The point is to manage to control the proportion of Type F Foods, which are those that increase glucose and insulin needs, which is why we put on weight.

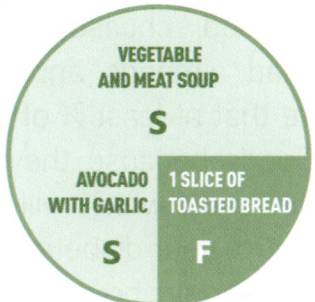 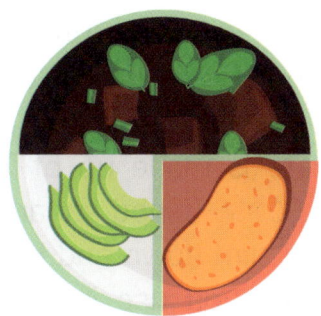

Excessive consumption of **Type F Foods** (FATTENING – Act as a FOE (ENEMIES) for the control of diabetes) is the main cause of overweight, obesity and most of the damage to diabetics. Type F Foods increase glucose (blood sugar) and excess glucose, in turn, is what causes both obesity and damage (blindness, amputations, kidney damage) in diabetic patients. That is why, in the 3x1 Diet, you can eat anything, but always making sure that no more than ¼ part of your plate is composed of Type F Foods.

Type F Foods include foods such as: bread, pasta, cookies, pizza, wheat, or corn flour, rice, beans ("frijoles" in Mexico), potatoes, yucca, sweet potatoes ("camote" in Mexico), plantains, tubers, cereals, fruits, fruit juices, milk, sweets, chocolates or sugar. Type F Foods are the ones that our body usually asks for the most and the ones that cause the most addiction, therefore your next step, before starting your 3x1 Diet, is to break the addiction or vice to Type F Foods, detoxifying your body from them. We will see in detail how to do this Type F Foods Detox later.

On the other hand, **Type S Foods** (SLIMMING – Helps SUPPORT the control of diabetes) are foods such as: beef, pork, chicken, turkey, fish, seafood, cheeses, eggs, vegetables, vegetable juices, salad, almonds, and nuts. While on the 3x1 Diet make sure that at least ¾ of your plate is made up of Type S Foods because they are GLUCOSE (blood sugar) REDUCING foods, which will help you slim down and help you control your diabetes. The foods you use in your 3x1 Diet should be combined according to your type of nervous system, which we will see in the next chapter.

Pathway to an Ultra-Powerful Metabolism

∞ **The 3x1 Diet helps us achieve METABOLIC BALANCE and restore metabolism.**
- The proportion of Type S Foods, which are slimming, and Type F Foods, which are FATTENING, are combined in the correct way.
- Type S Foods, should take ¾ parts of your food plate and Type F Foods should take only ¼ part of your food plate.
- The combination of foods in the 3x1 Diet should be made according to your type of nervous system, as will be discussed in the next chapter.

∞ Answer the following questions

1. Make a list of your favorite foods.
   Then, classify them by writing next to them whether they are Type S Foods or Type F Foods.

2. Observe your classified list, which type of foods do you consume more, Type S or Type F?

3. In what way do you think you could apply the 3x1 Diet to your breakfast, lunch and dinner to achieve your goals?

THE RIGHT NUTRITION BASED ON YOUR TYPE OF NERVOUS SYSTEM

Applying the correct nutrition according to the type of nervous system that is predominant in our body is vital in the process of restoring our metabolism.

By making this information available to all, mainly through MetabolismoTV, testimonials began pouring in from people all over the world who, being able to differentiate between whether their bodies had a primarily Excited or Passive Nervous System, were slimming down much faster, diabetics had their glucose levels lowered, and others reported enjoying a level of energy never experienced before.

We had reports of cases of people who for years had been suffering from insomnia (a problem mainly of the EXCITED) who, by changing their diet, had begun, for the first time in a long time, to sleep well and some were able to stop using antidepressant medications.

We noticed that when people had their diet modified based on the type of nervous system that was dominant in their bodies, they were able to slim down and had good results more quickly.

By adjusting the 3x1 Diet of overweight or obese diabetics to consider whether they had a predominantly Excited or Passive Nervous System, glucose levels were much better regulated, while the person lost excess fat at a faster rate. Adjusting the type of food to be consumed based on the type of nervous system, achieved exceptional results in making the metabolism more efficient.

A diet is about **food,** and food is what **fuels** your **metabolism**, just as the gasoline in your car FUELS your car's ENGINE. A diet deals only with the type of fuel in the body and the technology of metabolism deals with what happens inside the body when the cells must convert that combustible (food) into **energy** to survive.

Logic dictates that if you were having problems with your car's engine you would not try to solve it by improving the quality or type of gasoline you use as fuel.

A diet is to the metabolism as gasoline is to the engine of your car. There are cars whose engine uses a light fuel such as gasoline, while there are other cars that have heavier engines that use a denser fuel, such as diesel.

You cannot put gasoline in a diesel engine, nor can you put diesel fuel to an engine that uses gasoline, because they will be damaged. Each type of engine uses the appropriate fuel for that type of engine. The same thing happens with your body's metabolism because the diet (fuel) cannot be the same for everyone, because WE ARE NOT ALL THE SAME.

There can be no such thing as a "balanced diet" no matter how much we are told about it. We would have to ask ourselves, balanced for whom if we are not all the same? What may be an appropriate food for one may also be a poison for another, due to the biological individuality[78] of each one of us. Using the metabolism, we seek to restore and regulate the metabolic rate, so that nervous activity is neither overexcited nor shut down.

We seek to achieve METABOLIC BALANCE as much as possible where there is neither excess nor lack of nervous excitement. The closer we can get to achieve METABOLIC BALANCE, the better the overall health of our body will be.

As long as the nervous system undergoes drastic changes with over-excitement or lack of excitement, basically out of ignorance of the body's owner (you), the levels of stress hormones (cortisol, adrenaline) and hormones that manage the body's fat creation (insulin and glucagon) will keep your body on a roller coaster ride that will throw your metabolism out of control.

The body's nervous system needs to be controlled to restore metabolism. That starts with knowing what type of nervous system is dominant in your body and then, knowing what types of foods will help you balance your body's nervous system.

---

[78] biological individuality: differences between the bodies of different people due to hereditary factors that affect everything in the body, including blood type.

With metabolism technology, what we are primarily trying to restore is METABOLISM EFFICIENCY, and we do that by understanding what happens inside the body once you have ingested a certain food. Each type of food that is ingested has two possible effects on the body:

1. Provides the body with nutritional value based on its contribution of nutrients.

2. Causes an effect on the nervous and hormonal system, which influences the body's metabolism.

With the technology of metabolism, we look at the nutritional value of the food that is being used as combustible for the body's metabolism. In addition, we take into consideration the very important fact that each food has a different capacity to excite or calm the body's Autonomous Nervous System; and that this effect must be known and observed in order to regulate and make the metabolism more efficient.

Therefore, the nutrition for both types of nervous system is different. Those with a Passive Nervous System like me, Frank Suárez, have more carnivorous bodies, we need to eat red meat often and we benefit from a higher fat intake.

Those who have bodies with an Excited Nervous System, like my wife Elizabeth, gain weight when they eat fat or red meat. So, the recommendations for eating according to your nervous system type are as follows:

Recommended Foods According to the Type of Nervous System

Excited Nervous System	Passive Nervous System
Diet with more abundance of vegetables and salads.	More carnivorous diet.
Moderate consumption of white and low-fat proteins: chicken, turkey, and fish.	Red meats, pork and more fatty fish such as salmon, tuna, and sardines.
Small portions of low-fat cheeses.	Larger portions of cheeses.
Eggs cooked in water, in omelet or scrambled (not fried in oil).	Eggs prepared in any form (including fried eggs).
Consumption of an abundance of salads and vegetables.	Vegetables and salad are recommended to be combined with meats and seafood.
Low-fat and low sugar yogurt.	Yogurt low in sugar and carbohydrates.
The ideal dressing is olive oil and lemon or vinegar. Avoid creamy dressings; they have fat.	The ideal dressing is olive oil and lemon or vinegar. Avoid sugary dressings such as "Thousand Island".
Restricting sugar, fruits, sweets, bread, and flours, such as wheat or corn.	Restricting sugar, fruits, sweets, bread, and flours, such as wheat or corn.
Use of whole salt such as Himalayan, sea or Celtic salt.	Use of whole salt such as Himalayan, sea or Celtic salt.
Drinking coffee on a regular basis is good for you.	Moderate use of coffee.
3x1 Diet, low in Type F Foods = FATTENING (Refined Carbohydrates)	3x1 Diet, low in Type F Foods = FATTENING (Refined Carbohydrates)

If you happen to have an Excited Nervous System body, an example of a 3x1 Diet dish that would be recommended for your type of nervous system would be a combination of foods that are low in fat with no red meat or pork, like the illustration on the right.

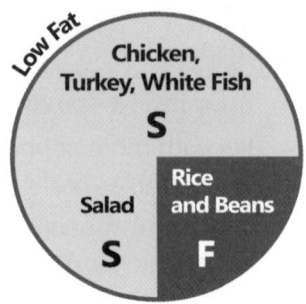

The body with an Excited Nervous System is a tense body, which tends to suffer from high blood pressure, muscle tension (especially in the shoulders, neck and lower back and legs), a certain difficulty with digestion (especially when eating very late at night) and often has a poor quality of sleep or suffers from insomnia.

A type of body where the Excited Nervous System, which is the system that the body activates when it must defend itself, is in a constant state of alertness and tension, as if preparing to fight or flee. When the Excited Nervous System is predominant in a person's body, the senses (sight, smell, hearing) are more sensitive or developed and the person sometimes sees, smells, or hears things that are difficult for others to perceive.

The Excited Nervous System puts the body in a state of alert! This system is the one that is activated when it is necessary to defend oneself, fight, run, act quickly, such as when there is an emergency, perceive danger or in some other way get into motion and action.

We are not talking, at any point about the personality, attitude, habits, or behavior of a person, only about the body, a living organism distinct from the person. Therefore, we must feed it with the nutrients that will calm it down. Fats and red meat are very stimulating and will not help you with that. In the next chapter we will see what other things, besides changing your diet, we can do to calm the Excited Nervous System.

If it turns out that you have a Passive Nervous System, it means that you have one of those privileged body types that eats everything and that everything goes down well. Those of us who have a Passive Nervous System "can even eat stones" and we digest everything well. We can eat late at night and still digest it well. We are deep sleepers and what really makes us gain weight is bread, flour, and sugar.

For those of us with a Passive Nervous System, what makes us gain weight are refined carbohydrates, such as rice, and even most fruits, which are excessively sweet due to their high fructose content (except strawberries or apples, which are the least sweet).

Among the people with a Passive Nervous System, hypothyroidism reigns, and it becomes important to avoid foods that interfere with the thyroid, such as soy. The Passive Nervous System is a carnivorous body that needs to eat red meat (beef, pork) because red meat excites the nervous system and that is precisely what the body of a passive needs, it needs excitement to balance itself.

As passive people, we can eat any meats, even if it is white meat, but we should always make sure we eat enough red meat. The reason is that red meat has a high content of natural substances called purines[79] which are very energizing substances, which do the passive a lot of good, in terms of helping our metabolism to produce a greater amount of energy.

On the contrary, for those with an Excited Nervous System, the purines in red meat cause an excessive additional stimulation that unbalances their metabolism and even makes them gain weight. The overstimulation that red meat and fat can cause to the body of an excited person, reduces the metabolism's energy.

If you happen to have a body with a Passive Nervous System, an example of a 3x1 Diet plate that would be recommended for your type of nervous system would be a combination of foods that are higher in red meat, pork or fatty

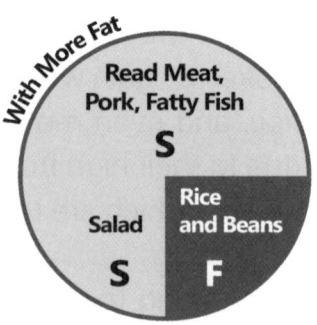

---

[79] purines: natural substances contained in DNA (deoxyribonucleic acid), which is the primary storage of hereditary genetic information in all living beings. When purines are used inside the cells, uric acid is produced. Excess uric acid, especially in those with an Excited Nervous System, can produce the inflammatory arthritic type of condition called gout. Foods that are high in purines have an exciting and stimulating effect on the nervous system, as well as causing constriction (narrowing that partially closes capillaries), which can raise blood pressure. Some foods with a high purine content are anchovies, crustaceans, sardines, meat, spinach and mushrooms.

fish (salmon, tuna) like the illustration on the right.

The body that has a Passive Nervous System needs food with more fat than the body with an Excited Nervous System. In fact, for those of us with a PASSIVE system, fat is not what makes us gain weight as it happens to the EXCITED ones. For the PASSIVE, what quickly makes us gain weight is bread, flour, sweets and refined carbohydrates.

It is important that this type of nutrition becomes a way of life for you. Many people start eating according to their nervous system type and begin to feel full of energy, can rest, and see that they are slimming down. Then they get the false idea that their type of nervous system has changed, for example, from EXCITED to PASSIVE, and they go back to eating fats or foods that excite the nervous system. This is a mistake and damages the progress they have made so far. If your predominant type of nervous system is EXCITED, know that you must adopt the correct type of nutrition according to your nervous system as a lifestyle.

Pathway to an Ultra-Powerful Metabolism

☞ **It is important to eat correctly according to our type of nervous system to restore your metabolism.**
- The nutrition recommended for people with an Excited Nervous System is lower in fat, white protein, abundant in vegetables and salad, and low in refined carbohydrates.

- The nutrition recommended for people with a Passive Nervous System is higher in red meat, with more fat and very low in refined carbohydrates.
- Nutrition according to our type of nervous system should be adopted as a way of life so as not to harm our nervous system and metabolism again.

👀 Answer the following questions

1. Describe what your nutrition should be like, according to your type of nervous system.

2. Make a list of the foods you should avoid eating according to your type of nervous system.

3. Specify which Type of Nervous System, Excited or Passive, would benefit each of the following combinations of the 3x1 Diet.

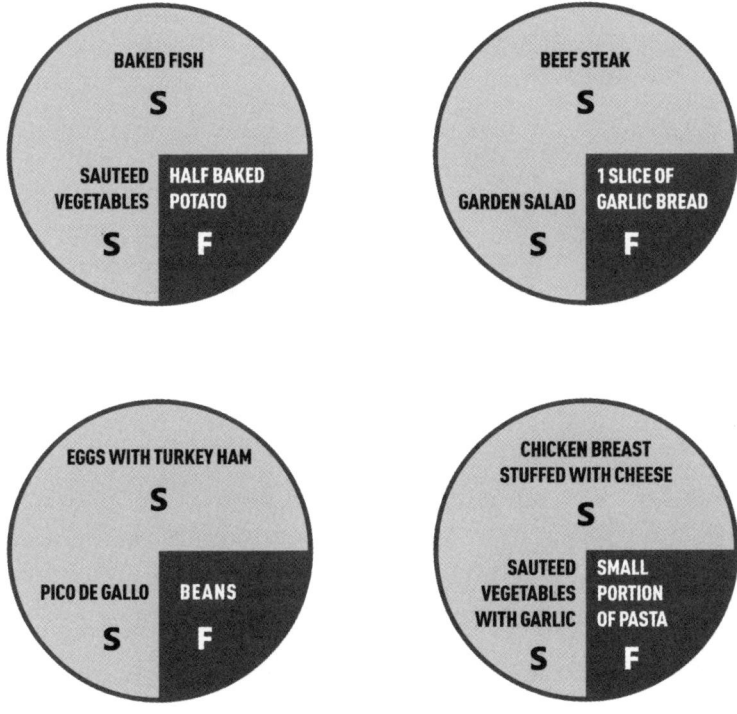

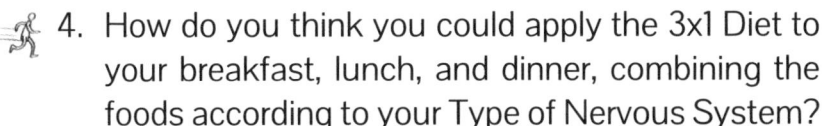 4. How do you think you could apply the 3x1 Diet to your breakfast, lunch, and dinner, combining the foods according to your Type of Nervous System?

How To Calm The Nervous System

Once you have taken the test to determine your type of nervous system in the previous chapters, you will know that, if you answered -YES- to any of the five test questions, your body has an Excited Nervous System. If you answered -NO- to all five test questions, your body has a Passive Nervous System.

After having helped hundreds of thousands of people slim down and improve their metabolism and health at NaturalSlim, I can tell you, without a doubt, that knowing whether your body is an Excited or Passive Nervous System is one of the most important things you can accomplish, because it will allow you to properly choose the types of foods that will benefit your body the most.

Just as there are cars whose engine only run on gasoline (a light fuel) and other cars or trucks whose engine only run-on diesel fuel (a heavy fuel), so too are human bodies different.

The main error of traditional nutrition is to consider that there must be a "balanced diet" that would be the best and most adequate for all people. For the traditional schools of nutrition, we are all the same and there are no genetic or hereditary differences as to the type of food that is beneficial for each person. It is a fixed idea[80] of the

---

[80] fixed idea: a decision or thought about something, which is unchangeable.

nutrition authorities who are unaware of the very important subject of METABOLISM and who want to force us all to consume the same type of food. This is a serious mistake and the increasing rates of obesity and diabetes prove it. A main reason why the NaturalSlim centers have been so successful and are already operating in eight countries is precisely because we learned to recognize that EVERYONE IS DIFFERENT therefore nutrition and food selection cannot be the same for everyone.

There are people with Excited Nervous System whose body does not tolerate or does not benefit from red meat or fat and depend on light foods such as white meats (chicken, turkey, fish), low fat foods and having an abundant consumption of vegetables and salads.

On the other hand, there are some of us who, by staying on a diet low in red meat or fat, simply become weaker because we have a Passive Nervous System. In other words, food that is good for one person can be poison for another precisely because we are ALL DIFFERENT.

Interestingly, I have observed that almost all couples are composed of an EXCITED with a PASSIVE. This is not a general rule and has its exceptions, but it certainly is a pattern that we have observed in most couples. When the husband eats everything because he has "a stone stomach" and digests everything well, his wife has a delicate stomach or vice versa. When the husband sleeps soundly and nothing wakes him up, the wife wakes up at any slight noise, spends the night awake suffering from insomnia, and wakes up tired.

Having had the opportunity to observe thousands of couples who attended NaturalSlim to slim down, control diabetes or regain their energy allowed us to realize that, in a great majority of cases, the opposite types of nervous system (EXCITED vs. PASSIVE) attract each other, as if they were the opposite poles of negative and positive of a magnet. Therefore, we know that, in the vast majority of cases, whatever is the right nutrition for the wife (if she has an Excited Nervous System will also be poor nutrition for the husband who has a Passive Nervous System.

Now that you know that WE ARE ALL NOT CREATED EQUAL and that we all have different food needs according to the type of nervous system we inherited, you should also know that I have discovered that major health problems mainly affect people who have an Excited Nervous System.

The Excited Nervous System of the body is designed only for the vital functions of "fight or flight", to cope with the dangers and threats that the environment throws at us and everything has to do with STRESS.

That is why, when a person has an Excited Nervous System, the STRESS accumulated in the nervous system begins to cause digestive problems, poor sleep quality, constipation, high blood pressure, fluid retention, thyroid problems, back pain, arthritis and even cancer, if the person does not manage to calm his or her Excited Nervous System.

Over the past twenty years of helping hundreds of thousands of people at NaturalSlim I have been able to confirm that the most serious metabolism and health problems always seem to be caused by STRESS ACCUMULATED in the Excited Nervous System of a person's body.

So, if by taking the test you turned out to have an Excited Nervous System, this information will help you calm your nervous system so that you can improve your metabolism and health to achieve your goals. If after answering -NO- to the five questions in the test you turned out to have, like me, Frank Suárez, a Passive Nervous System, then it is up to you to learn this information so you can help your partner or loved ones who are being affected by an Excited Nervous System. I have observed in thousands of cases that there does not seem to be any health condition that cannot be improved when you apply these techniques that I will share with you to CALM THE Excited Nervous System.

Your brain works like a computer that in an automatic and continuous way (it works twenty-four hours a day and seven days a week) regulates and controls EVERYTHING that goes on in your body including the creation of energy, which is what we call metabolism.

The brain is part of your body's nervous system and from there it regulates your heart rate, digestion, sleep quality, sexuality, hormones, detoxification, your mood and all the other multiple systems that make up your body. When EXCESS STRESS has accumulated in the nervous system, the EXCITED side of the nervous system remains more active and the function of the PASSIVE side that we all have is reduced.

PASSIVE Nervous System

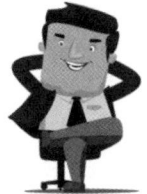

State of Relaxation
and Rest

EXCITED Nervous System

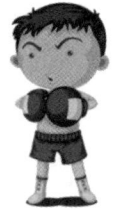

State of Alert
Ready to Fight or Flee

The Excited Nervous System, when overstimulated and STRESS builds up, can produce an incredible variety of unpleasant manifestations and bizarre health conditions for which your doctor will have no solution. These are conditions and diseases such as: obesity, accumulation of abdominal fat, poor digestion, poor sleep quality, arthritis, bone loss, high blood pressure (hypertension), constipation, hair loss when combing your hair, back pain, depression, irritability, anxiety, attention deficit, insomnia, not enough restful sleep, poor circulation, thyroid problems, diabetes, loss of interest in your sexual partner, impotence in men, and even cancer.

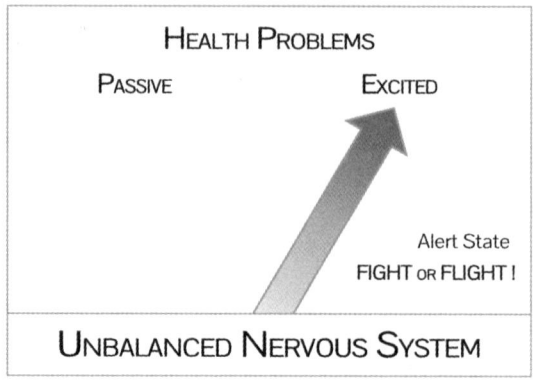

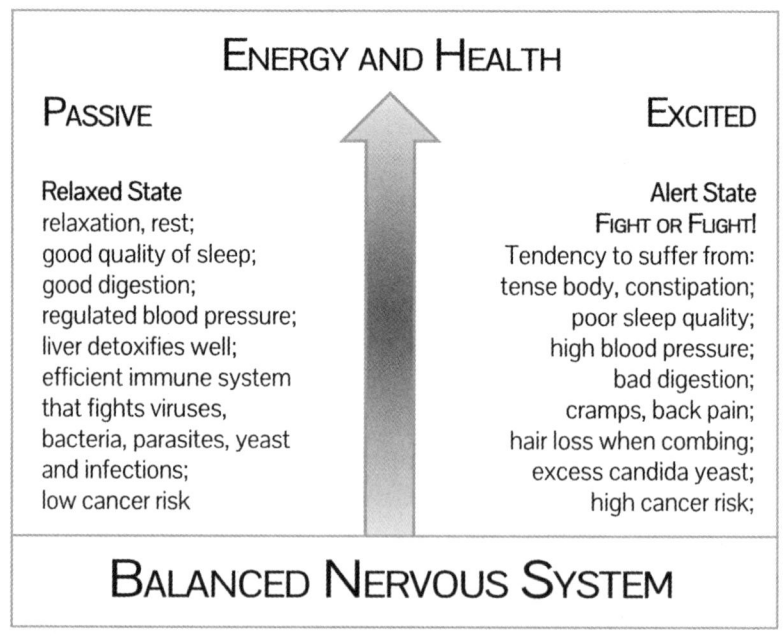

If you happen to have an Excited Nervous System know that to control your metabolism, and improve your body's health and energy, it is vital to CALM THE Excited Nervous System.

The different actions I have discovered that work to calm the Excited Nervous System are explained in my free educational videos on MetabolismoTV on YouTube. The information on everything you can do to calm your body's Excited Nervous System is contained in these short educational videos.

If you watch these videos I recommend below and follow each of these recommendations I make, you will see that you will slim down easily, improve your quality of sleep, improve your energy level, and even improve your emotional state. When you apply the knowledge of how to calm the Excited Nervous System you are actually bringing your body to a point of greater BALANCE. By doing this, your METABOLISM and energy level can only improve.

In the NaturalSlim centers we have been able to prove with hundreds of thousands of people helped, that all deficient health conditions (obesity, diabetes, depression) or chronic illnesses (arthritis, high blood pressure, cancer) only occur when there is an imbalance in the NERVOUS SYSTEM which is the system that controls the body and metabolism. By adjusting your lifestyle and consuming foods according to your type of nervous system, your health will improve in no time.

The videos I recommend you watch on MetabolismoTV to educate yourself on how to calm the nervous system to improve your metabolism, your energy, and your health are the following:

Episode #	MetabolismoTV Videos to Calm the Nervous System
	Episode Title (Video)
1043	Tricks to Calm the Nervous System
828	Vegetable Juices Save Lives
951	Connection to Earth
979	Breathe and Slim Down
1281	Magnesium to the Rescue
1196	How Much Magnesium Should I Take
1340	Potassium. How much? Why?

As we saw in the videos, we need to hydrate according to our body size, have the correct nutrition for our nervous system, do deep breathing, land connection, sunbathe and provide our body with the potassium and magnesium it needs through nutrition, supplementation and drinking vegetable juices.

If you haven't watched the videos, I recommend you stop here and do so. The information that I present in each video is vital for you to ensure your success and restore your metabolism.

By following the recommendations I have made in this book such as hydrating your body properly, doing the 3x1 Diet to reduce Type F (FATTENING) foods and educating yourself about thyroid problems, candida yeast, foods that are aggressors of your body (which we will see later) and many other recommendations I have shared with you, for sure you will improve your metabolism, your energy level and your health.

You CANNOT fail to apply this knowledge to improve your body simply because what I have shared with you in this book are TRUTHS. TRUTHS ALWAYS PRODUCE GOOD RESULTS just as LIES always produce BAD RESULTS.

I invite you to stay informed about the latest discoveries by subscribing for free to my educational video channel MetabolismoTV on YouTube. Remember, **The Truth... Always Triumphs!**

About Attention Deficit and Hyperactivity Disorder

Unfortunately, many children are diagnosed with the fashionable mental illnesses, "Attention Deficit" or "Hyperactivity", supposed mental illnesses that are based on opinions and for which there is no reliable scientific proof (laboratory analysis, X-rays, electrocardiogram, etc.). You should also know that the theory of "brain chemical imbalances" proposed by the promoters of these diseases has never been proven.

I am afraid that the victims of these psychiatric diagnostics [81] are often children who for hereditary reasons have an Excited Nervous System and that their parents, out of unawareness, allow them to have a diet that contains stimulating substances such as sugar, sweets, fat and salt. In some cases, these children are

---

[81] diagnostics: the word diagnostic is formed from *diag-* which means "through" and *gnosis* which means "knowledge". A diagnostic is a decision that a physician or health professional makes based on his knowledge of the condition or disease and what he observes in the patient.

given carbonated soft drinks (Coca-Cola, Sprite, etc.) which are actually "sweet liquids", since one of these soft drinks contains up to three tablespoons of sugar.

It is sad that we must end up drugging our children with psychotropic medications such as Ritalin, Adderall, Concerta and others, which are equivalent to street medications such as cocaine, simply because we do not know what kind of nourishment would calm their Excited Nervous System. When the nervous system is too EXCITED, the person or child cannot focus their attention because the body is having a nervous breakdown.

If you have children with this type of attention deficit or hyperactivity problems please check their diet and other factors that can produce an EXCITED state of the nervous system such as: candida albicans yeast infection (candidiasis), gluten intolerance (the protein in wheat, bread, pizza), allergies [82] to colorants or preservatives, heavy metal poisoning, pesticide contamination, hormonal problems, high sugar diet or other real medical, nutritional or environmental causes that could be hidden by a diagnosis that is not based on verifiable scientific evidence such as attention deficit or hyperactivity.

You can learn more about the real possible causes of behavioral or learning problems at Dr. Mary Ann Block's Web site, www.blockcenter.com. You can also learn

---

[82] allergies: an allergy is a specific response of the immune system, which is the defense system in our body. It is a specific reaction to certain foods or substances that develops an immediate reaction such as itching, mucus, headache, or other manifestations.

about parental rights at www.cchrint.org (English) or www.cchrlatam.org (Spanish).

Pathway to an Ultra-Powerful Metabolism

∞ The Excited Nervous System can be calmed by doing the following:
- Hydrate correctly, by using the formula for calculating glasses of water according to your body weight.
- To follow the correct diet, according to your type of nervous system.
- Breathe deeply, as shown in the videos.
- Grounding to discharge the electrical overload of your nervous system.
- Sunbathing, as explained in the videos.
- Drink fresh vegetable juices.
- Supplement the body properly with the magnesium and potassium it needs.
- Avoid toxic people.

∞ Answer the following questions
1. Describe the manifestations that can be caused by having an Unbalanced Nervous System.

2. **Assuming you have an Excited Nervous System, what specific actions** have you decided to take to calm it down?

REFINED CARBOHYDRATES DETOX

Now that you know your body's nervous system type, EXCITED or PASSIVE, you can start eating according to the 3x1 Diet ratio to restore your metabolism. However, there is one obstacle you must overcome if you want to ensure success in your new lifestyle.

As we saw, Type F Foods (FATTENING – Act as a FOE (ENEMIES) for the control of diabetes) which are refined carbohydrates, and starches, among others, have the power to cause addiction. We have been abusing the consumption of Type F Foods for so long that most people suffer from a very strong addiction to these foods. So strong is the need for carbonated soft drinks, chocolates, sweets, bread, tortillas, or any other Type F Foods, that they simply must consume one of these foods daily, otherwise they feel they are missing something or cannot function. If they try not to consume them, they feel very anxious, and their emotional state is negatively affected.

If you feel anxiety or a strong craving for a specific food daily, it is a given that you are experiencing an addictive relationship with that food. What happens is that when we consume an excess of refined carbohydrates the brain increases its production of serotonin[83]. Serotonin works as a tranquilizer and for a period we feel relaxed, and anxiety is removed. So, the body becomes addicted to the effect of serotonin and, when we are under stress or anxious, it asks for Type F Foods to feel this effect.

If we do not handle this addiction to Type F Foods, you will hardly be successful in your attempt to live the 3x1 Diet lifestyle, simply because your body will not allow you to do so, by demanding that you supply it with the foods you are addicted to.

So, we must detoxify the body from its addiction to Type F Foods. Know that it is important to withdraw from the addiction gradually, so as not to cause a crisis to the body. You should also know that during the process of detoxification from refined carbohydrates you may experience unpleasant physical reactions, as happens when we try to break the addiction to any kind of substance. To learn more about how our body creates dependence to refined carbohydrates, I recommend you watch Episode #829 on MetabolismoTV.

In order not to cause a stress crisis to the body, we start with a body preparation day in which we begin by consuming large amounts of water. Also, during this day, you can consume Type F Foods, but in smaller quantities than you usually do. This way we create the necessary environment in the body to break the addiction.

---

[83] serotonin: a substance produced by the brain that has an antidepressant effect and is considered responsible for causing a good mood.

The following day, our 48 HOUR DETOXIFICATION PERIOD begins, in which we will only consume proteins; that is, only meats, cheeses and eggs, according to our type of nervous system. So, for the next 48 hours we will eliminate the consumption of any refined carbohydrates (bread, rice, tortillas, potatoes, pasta, sugar, etc.) and we will also eliminate the consumption of natural carbohydrates (vegetables, salads, etc.).

During these two days of withdrawal, we are looking to break the addiction by removing ALL sources of carbohydrates from the body. So, during the days of total carbohydrate withdrawal, you consume no salads, no vegetables, no juices, no sweeteners, no sugar or sugar substitutes in coffee, no milk, or anything that contains carbohydrates. Likewise, when cooking your proteins, you should do so without vegetables (such as onions, etc.) or sauces, as these are carbohydrates.

Only meats such as chicken, turkey, fish, beef, pork; cheese and eggs are consumed. You should choose which ones to consume according to your type of nervous system. For example, if you have an Excited Nervous System, you should consume white, low-fat meats, eggs that are not fried and low-fat cheeses, such as fresh cheese called country cheese or panela cheese. If, on the contrary, your nervous system is Passive, you can consume all types of meats and cheeses, even if they contain fat.

It is important that during these two days you do not experience hunger. You should consume different combinations of meats, cheeses, and eggs, according to your type of nervous system, but without limiting the quantity. During these two days, if you feel hungry between meals, it is okay to snack, but only meats, cheeses, or eggs. You should feel satisfied and not go hungry, as it will cause additional stress to the body if you do so.

Just as on the preparatory day, water consumption is vital during these two days of detoxification from refined carbohydrates. The body will be under some level of stress during these two detox days as you are taking away the foods you are addicted to. So, it will produce cortisol, which is the stress hormone. Drinking water will help remove this hormone and calm the hormonal system.

A great help that can be used is to consume a daily dose of one to two teaspoons of a magnesium-based product, which we distribute at NaturalSlim, called MagicMag. The mineral magnesium has a relaxing and anti-stress effect, both on the nervous system and on the body's hormonal system. So, it will help you detoxify your body, without too much suffering. The MagicMag magnesium offered by NaturalSlim centers is a more absorbable magnesium than the other seven types of magnesium. If you cannot get it in your country, you can use any other type of magnesium, except magnesium oxide, which happens to be the worst absorbed. If you can find MagicMag, all the better, as we have seen that when this magnesium is used, relaxation is more complete, even sleep quality is improved and insulin resistance is reduced.

It is very common that during this period of withdrawal from refined carbohydrates you experience reactions such as migraine, headache, itchy skin, vaginal discharge, diarrhea or muscle aches. What is happening is that your body is severely infected with the candida albicans yeast, which we will discuss in detail later. This yeast is totally dependent on carbohydrates for its maintenance. Without carbohydrates the yeast has no way to survive. Therefore, when there is a candida yeast infection and all carbohydrates are removed from the diet, the yeast is left without its food and begins to die and rot inside the body due to lack of food. When it rots, the body fills with the acids and toxins released by the yeast and all these manifestations occur. Usually, the manifestations do not last more than a day, but I must say that they can be quite unpleasant.

To recap, the entire Refined Carbohydrate Detox process has a three-day duration: a preparatory day and then two days of detoxification without consuming any carbohydrates. In addition to eliminating cravings, desires, or addiction to Type F Foods, the detoxification process prepares your hormonal system to burn fat by reducing the production of the insulin hormone (hormone that makes you fat) and increasing the production of the hormone glucagon (hormone that makes you slim). So, after completing your detoxification process from refined carbohydrates you are ready to begin your 3x1 Diet style eating and ensure your success.

Pathway to an Ultra-Powerful Metabolism

∞ **The Refined Carbohydrate Detox process helps ensure success in the metabolism restoration process.**
- The process lasts three days: the preparatory day and 48 hours of detoxification.
- During the two days of detox only meats, cheeses, and eggs are consumed, depending on the type of nervous system.
- There is no limit to the amount of food consumed during these two days and you should not go hungry.

∞ **Answer the following questions**
1. Make a list of the specific foods that you can consume during the two days of detoxification, according to your type of nervous system.

2. Describe what foods you will make for breakfast, lunch and dinner during your 48-hour detoxification that apply to your type of nervous system.

SLEEP BETTER OR FAIL

There are some truths about metabolism that life experience has taught us that if ignored will cause us to fail to achieve our goals. To achieve an Ultra-Powerful Metabolism, you must be willing to "sleep better or fail".

Working in the NaturalSlim centers with hundreds of thousands of people to help them overcome slow metabolism, we discovered a truth that can be summarized in the following invariable rule: **you will only have as good energy and health as the quality of sleep you get each night.**

Those of us who have a Passive Nervous System rarely have difficulty enjoying deep, restful sleep. However, among those with an excited nervous system, it is quite common that they do not enjoy optimal sleep quality. When the excited nervous system is overstimulated, the body enters its alert phase and prepares to "fight or flee," which in turn deactivates the Passive Nervous System, which is what allows us to enjoy a refreshing and restful sleep.

People whose bodies have an Excited Nervous System too often sleep in an interrupted manner, with one or more interruptions of sleep to make trips to the bathroom to urinate and having a shallow sleep that causes them to wake up and lose sleep at even the slightest external noise. When sleep is not very deep and there are interruptions during sleep, the person does not achieve a restful sleep and wakes up still feeling tired in the morning. At that moment when you wake up in the morning, open your eyes and feel a deep tiredness, know that your metabolism is in bad shape.

The less hours of deep and restful sleep a person gets, the worse the results will be with their metabolism improvement project. To slim down, to control diabetes, even to regain energy and health, it is very important to achieve a period of restorative sleep. Getting a good, deep, refreshing, and restful sleep for enough hours each night (at least seven hours) is vital to improve metabolism and body health.

To some people who ignore these truths about the importance of getting sleep to restore the body's energy, it seems to them that sleep is a "waste of time". These are people with very busy lives and work schedules, so some would like to get as little sleep as possible to "make the most of their time". Most of them are people who have lived for so many years accustomed to experiencing severe daily stress, plus the lack of good sleep, that they mistakenly consider it completely normal to have interrupted sleep of poor quality or a period of sleep that is too short.

The reality is that one can get used to almost any situation in life. The proof of this is that almost all of us have met a married couple who live their lives fighting and criticizing each other; however, they have become accustomed to their infernal relationship and already consider it normal. The same thing happens with poor sleep quality. The person can become accustomed to long nights of interrupted sleep, to having few hours of sleep and to carrying a continuous tiredness that forces them to consume stimulants such as coffee or cigarettes to stay alert.

When the nervous system remains in a state of excitement, the person is unable to reconcile a restful sleep and tiredness accumulates. To sleep, the Passive Nervous System must first be activated. If this PASSIVE system is not activated, the state of nervous excitement will not allow a repairing sleep to be achieved.

To understand how important the subject of sleep is, it is very helpful to understand the cycle[84] of life. A cycle is a sequence of actions that occur one after the other and at the end of the sequence occur again in the same order. For example, plants are born, grow and die. We are born, we grow and one day we will die. To this sequence of being born, growing, and dying is called the cycle of life and no plant or living organism can escape this cycle. Everything that is alive must at some point be born, grow and die.

---

[84] cycle: a series of phases, states or actions that occur one after the other and, at the end of the sequence, occur again in the same order. Some examples are the menstrual cycle, the solar cycle, the cycle of the seasons.

In fact, all the cells in your body are also part of the cycle of life. That is why every cell that makes up your body had to be born, then it grew, and finally it will end up dying.

The human body, which is part of living organisms, is also being part of the cycle of life so your body is in a continuous activity of birth, growth and cell death that keep you in a continuous process of renewal. The skin your body has today is no longer the skin you were born with, because every six weeks your body has renewed and replaced the cells that create your skin.

There is another very important cycle in which our human body participates, which is called the circadian cycle[85]. The circadian cycle is the body's internal clock. You know that the sun rises in the morning, the day goes by, the sun sets, and the night comes in. In the same way in our body, we have an internal clock, which controls certain daily functions of our body, especially our ability to sleep, which is called the circadian cycle.

This cycle controls the hours of production of many hormones in the body, especially the production of the cortisol hormone, which is the stress hormone, and the production of the melatonin hormone, which is the hormone that helps us sleep.

---

[85] circadian cycle: the word circadian comes from the Latin word *circa* which means "around" and from the Latin word *dies* which means "day". So, the circadian cycle refers to the changes that occur to living beings at regular time intervals and that are repeated daily.

The production of the cortisol hormone starts to be activated around six o'clock in the morning. This hormone has to be activated because it prepares us to give us energy to start the day. Therefore, it increases its production from six o'clock in the morning and at about eleven o'clock in the morning it reaches its peak. Then it lowers its production so as not to cause so much excitement and allow us to rest at night. Its lowest point of production is between ten and eleven o'clock at night.

On the other hand, the melatonin hormone stops its production in the morning, so that we can wake up, and starts to increase its production around nine o'clock at night. The melatonin hormone helps in many processes in the body, but mainly it is the hormone that makes us sleepy, to ensure that we sleep and that the body can carry out all its repair processes. The production of the melatonin hormone depends very much on the amount of light we are exposed to. That is why, when night falls and the sunlight goes down, we feel ourselves getting sleepy naturally. The body starts producing melatonin around nine o'clock at night and its peak production is between midnight and three o'clock in the morning.

This sleep cycle can be affected by our habits. For example, you may have noticed that, if you choose to stay awake after ten to eleven o'clock at night, there comes a time when you are sleep deprived and then you are wide awake. This happens because you have stopped the production of the melatonin hormone because you are getting too much light and have forced the body to produce more cortisol hormone to have energy and stay awake.

So, the most recommended time to go to sleep is between nine and eleven o'clock at night, because in this period is when there is less cortisol production in your body and the production of the melatonin hormone has started to help you sleep.

It is important to know that the sleeping process and the sleep are an integral part of the body's renewal process. That is why a person who sleeps too few hours or has poor quality interrupted sleep ages faster. Note that if you had a bad night where you were unable to get a good night's sleep, you will clearly feel the difference in the body's energy level and mental clarity the next day.

Scientific literature shows that poor quality or little sleep has a very negative impact on the nervous and hormonal system. We already know that stress makes you fat because stress forces your body to produce an excess of the stress hormone called cortisol which in turn increases your glucose (blood sugar) levels and makes you put on weight, especially in the abdominal area.

If you do not get a good night's sleep, your cortisol levels stay too high and that will prevent you from slimming down. Anyone who has had a bad night's sleep, if they experiment with taking a glucose measurement with a glucometer, will find that their fasting glucose levels often rise above 100 milligrams per deciliter. A person who sleeps well and does not suffer from diabetes will always have fasting glucose levels below 100 mg/dl.

So, to achieve an Ultra-Powerful Metabolism you must find a way to get restorative sleep to help you renew your body.

If you are having a period of little restorative sleep, interrupted or of few hours, it would be convenient for you to apply all the recommendations that we saw in the chapter entitled HOW TO CALM THE NERVOUS SYSTEM and the MetabolismoTV videos on the subject. We have already tested these recommendations with thousands of people, and I guarantee you that they work.

There are also other recommendations that will help you avoid overstimulation of the nervous system to prevent you from getting a restful sleep. These are some of those recommendations:

1. Do your best to find your AGGRESSOR FOODS with the help of a glucometer. Consuming AGGRESSOR FOODS causes an overstimulation of the Excited Nervous System, and this will affect the quality of your sleep. You will find out how to do this in a later chapter.

2. Make sure you sleep in a completely dark room. Light will make it difficult for you to get good quality sleep. You can also use a sleep mask to cover your eyes and help you fall asleep.

3. Avoid noises or noisy environments while you sleep. You can get earplugs that are placed in your ears to block sound and help you sleep without sleep interruptions from noise.

4. Avoid watching TV or working with your mobile phone or computer until an hour before bedtime. These electronic devices emit the so-called "blue light" that stimulates the Excited Nervous System and affects your quality of sleep.

5. I also recommend that when you go to sleep turn off your home's Wi-Fi internet and leave your mobile phone as far away as possible from the head of the bed, so that the electromagnetic waves do not overexcite your nervous system. The damage that electromagnetic waves do to the human body is scientifically proven. You can watch Episode #1227 of MetabolismoTV where I explain this topic more extensively.

6. A hot bath relaxes the body and therefore activates the Passive system which is the one that allows you to sleep.

7. Reading a good book before going to bed will help you sleep. Be sure to read it in a printed book rather than on a computer or electronic tablet to avoid "blue light" stimulation.

8. Also, whenever possible, remember to go to bed at the right time, taking advantage of your body's internal clock and the production of the melatonin hormone around nine to eleven o'clock at night. This will prevent your body from producing more of the cortisol hormone after hours and help you get a restorative night's sleep.

To achieve an Ultra-Powerful Metabolism, it is essential to get a relaxing and restful sleep. By following these recommendations, you will have the opportunity to activate your body's Passive Nervous System which is the one that guarantees a good quality of sleep. Sleeping well will prevent you from failing in your attempts to achieve your goals.

Pathway to an Ultra-Powerful Metabolism

👀 **Having a truly restful sleep is vital for maintaining health and restoring metabolism.**
- While we sleep, all the body's renewal processes take place and prevent us from aging.
- Sleeping badly causes us to wake up with an excess of glucose in our blood, which makes us put on weight and affects our metabolism.

👀 **Answer the following questions**
1. Describe what are your current common habits when you go to sleep.

2. How many hours of sleep do you get on a regular basis? Do you sleep deeply, or do you have many interruptions in your sleep during the night?

3. Describe what actions you will take to ensure that you get a truly restorative sleep and that you sleep at least seven hours a day.

Candida Albicans Yeast

One of the major causes of slow metabolism is infection of the body with the candida albicans yeast. The candida albicans yeast is one of more than 150 species of yeast that inhabit the human body. It is so named because this yeast is white in color. The word *candida* comes from the Latin word *candidus* which means bright white; and the word *albicans* comes from the Latin word *albus* which also means white.

All human beings have candida albicans yeast in our body, especially in the intestine, in the intestinal flora[86] and in women in addition in the vaginal flora. Under normal conditions, this yeast does not invade or cause disease. But if you neglect your diet by consuming an excess of refined carbohydrates, which is its favorite food, the candida yeast will reproduce aggressively in all parts of your body.

Since all human bodies are born with the candida yeast as part of their intestinal and vaginal flora, traditional medicine does not give much attention to this issue until the yeast has become so proliferated in the body that the condition called candidiasis occurs.

---

[86] flora: a collection of organisms such as bacteria, some viruses, parasites, and fungi that live inside the body on the walls of the intestine and the vagina in women. Most of these organisms help in different body processes and are harmless. However, some of them, under specific conditions, can cause damage to the body, such as, for example, the overgrowth of the candida yeast, which can invade the whole body and cause damage when a person consumes an excess of refined carbohydrates.

Traditional medicine considers that the candida yeast is only a problem for patients who are in a terminal state such as cancer and the acquired immune deficiency syndrome.

This is precisely why I called it THE SILENT EPIDEMIC because it is not paid attention to until it is already a serious condition, whereas long before it reaches this point, the candida albicans yeast is already causing devastation in the body and causing it to slow metabolism.

As I mentioned, the favorite food of the candida yeast is refined carbohydrates. Spending many years of your life consuming refined carbohydrates, you were unknowingly feeding this yeast, helping it to grow out of control. At this point, the yeast is already outgrowing the flora and traveling through the blood to all the organs of the body. It is already so well fed that it has reproduced ferociously, and your body's immune system cannot control it. This is called a systemic infection.

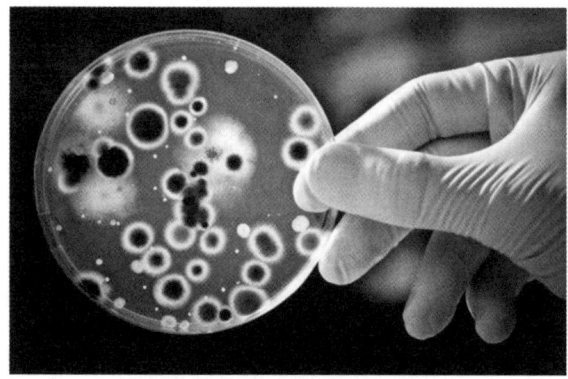

YEAST GROWING AND EXPANDING

People with systemic infections of this yeast always have a slow metabolism and fail to slim down under any diet or exercise regimen. If they do reduce their weight, they do so at such a slow rate that they are usually discouraged. This happens because the candida yeast produces 78 different toxins that create an acidic and very toxic environment inside the body that basically shuts down the metabolism.

The overgrowth of the candida yeast in the body is one of the main reasons why many people's weight loss efforts do not work for them. In my experience, nothing produces a more noticeable increase in metabolism and ability to slim down than doing a candida albicans yeast cleansing program.

Although laboratory tests to detect the levels of candida yeast in the body are very expensive and there really is no test that can truly measure the size and degree of the infection in a person's body, there is a very simple way to know how infected our body is with this yeast.

The toxics produced by the candida yeast in the body cause us to feel a series of symptoms or ailments for which traditional medicine has no explanation. According to how many of these symptoms we are suffering we can identify how infected we are with this yeast. Some of the most common manifestations or symptoms that people have due to the overgrowth of the candida yeast in their body are:

- ☐ acne
- ☐ allergy in humid environments
- ☐ allergies to some foods
- ☐ allergies to certain jewelry or metal jewelry
- ☐ continuous fatigue
- ☐ cystitis (urinary infections in women)
- ☐ constant or frequent diarrhea
- ☐ vaginal or burning pain when having sex
- ☐ headaches or migraines
- ☐ strong menstrual cramps
- ☐ muscle aches and pains
- ☐ constipation
- ☐ fatigue or weakness
- ☐ vaginal discharge or itching
- ☐ cold extremities
- ☐ stomach or intestinal gases in excess
- ☐ ear infections
- ☐ urinary tract infections
- ☐ irregularities or menstruation disorder
- ☐ irritability or depression
- ☐ itchy skin (especially at night or after showering)
- ☐ problems with digestive gases
- ☐ excessive skin dryness
- ☐ metal taste in the mouth
- ☐ rash or spot on the skin when sunbathing
- ☐ sensitivity to sunlight, watering eyes
- ☐ sensitivity to cigarette smell, perfumes o chemicals
- ☐ sinus

Of course, you could attribute many of these symptoms to a variety of other different CAUSES or MEDICAL CONDITIONS that your body has. It is precisely this confusion that has kept medicine in controversy about candida yeast infections in patients who are not terminally ill or near death, such as cancer patients.

Doctors find it difficult to believe that this candida yeast can cause so many manifestations like or the same as other known diseases, without being able to prove it. Meanwhile, the general population continues to suffer more and more every day from this SILENT EPIDEMIC.

I can understand the skepticism of doctors with this candida yeast topic, as they have been trained in the scientific discipline of accumulating evidence. However, the only thing I can tell you is that the hundreds of thousands of people who have done our yeast cleansing program give firm testimony (many of them which are signed) that after the yeast cleansing, more than half of their ailments (symptoms, pains, allergies, sinus, migraines, gases) disappeared along with the inflammation that their bodies had. All these people had a noticeable improvement in their metabolism once they did the NaturalSlim yeast cleansing program.

One important thing we have discovered, regarding the issues of candida yeast infections, is that the only thing that gets the yeast infection under control in the long run, is for the person to get EDUCATION that allows them to UNDERSTAND what their bad choices and poor lifestyle have been that led them to allow the candida yeast to take over their body. You cannot control something you do not understand! If you do not educate yourself and learn to adopt a lifestyle more conducive to health, there is no hope, because before long you will go back to eating an excess of bread, flours, rice, sweets, and other refined carbohydrates, which will surely allow the infection to take over again.

You should know that there is no possible way to eliminate 100% of the candida albicans yeast from the human body, because it is one of the normal resident organisms of the flora (intestinal and vaginal). What the candida yeast cleanse does is to REDUCE THE INVASIVE COLONY of yeast, to bring it to a point where the person's own immune system is able to control its invasive growth. Let's say we try to reduce the yeast colony from 100% to 10% and, if the person has been educated on how to prevent the infection from returning, we will have succeeded in restoring the metabolism and empowering the person.

There are three important factors that we consider vital when managing candida albicans yeast infection:

1. We prefer to use **a natural anti-fungal agent** rather than medications that can cause liver damage, as is the case with prescription anti-fungal medications (Nystatin, Diflucan, Amphotericin B, Candicindin and many others).

2. During the yeast cleanse, we want to provide the body with enough **good bacteria** (natural probiotics) so that the immune system is strengthened with a healthy intestinal flora.

3. We want to **educate the person** so that they do not continue to make the same mistakes in their food selection and lifestyle. Those judgment errors that allowed their metabolism to weaken and made their body fertile ground for a serious candida yeast infection. We are interested in managing the problem once and for all by improving the person's lifestyle and habits.

As I explained, we ALL have the candida yeast as a host in our body, because it is one of the normal inhabitants of the intestinal and vaginal flora. When there has been an excess consumption of refined carbohydrates and starches, the body becomes a breeding ground for yeast because it creates an environment for the candida yeast which is rich in its favorite nutrient, GLUCOSE. Once the yeast has continued to spread throughout the body, it becomes a systemic infection, or what doctors in the worst cases of their terminally ill patients would call "candidiasis." The yeast creates all sorts of symptoms such as allergies, fatigue, vaginal discharge, migraines, sinus, ear infections, skin infections and even depression.

At NaturalSlim we have had cases of people who were taking antidepressant medications for years, who had their depression episodes disappear once they finished their candida yeast cleanse. The highly toxic environment that candidiasis creates is sure to affect a person's brain, nervous system and emotional state. The only thing left for me to tell you is that

IT IS IN YOUR HANDS to do something about it. The time has come to restore your metabolism by giving it the toxin-free environment that your body needs to function properly.

Pathway to an Ultra-Powerful Metabolism

👀 **The candida yeast infection in the body affects the metabolism and general functions of the body.**
- Candida yeast feeds mainly on refined carbohydrates.
- When we eat refined carbohydrates in excess, the candida yeast spreads throughout the body causing a systemic infection.
- The candida albicans yeast produces 78 different toxins that create a highly acidic and toxic environment in the body that reduces metabolism.
- It is necessary to do a candida yeast cleanse to reduce the colony of this yeast in our body and restore metabolism.
- In addition to the cleanse, it is vital to moderate our consumption of Type F Foods to avoid a systemic infection of the yeast again.

👀 **Answer the following questions**
1. Write here all the manifestations you suffer from the list presented in this chapter. How many are there in total?

2. Of the symptoms you suffer from, are there any or some that you have suffered from for a long time? What have you done to improve them? What have been the results?

3. What decision have you made and what actions will you take regarding the prevalence of candida yeast in your body?

The Metabolism Control Center

We already know that energy creation occurs inside cells, specifically in the mitochondria. Yes, within the billions of cells in the body the combustion that drives metabolism occurs. Now, there is a gland in the body that controls or directs the activity of the body's metabolism. Whether we have an efficient and Ultra Powerful Metabolism, or a slow metabolism depends on the optimal functioning of this gland and the hormones it produces. This important gland is called the thyroid gland.

The thyroid gland is a gland that is located at the base of the neck and is shaped like a butterfly with open wings. From this gland the body's metabolism is controlled because the thyroid produces the T4 and T3 hormones, which are the hormones that determine how much OXYGEN enters the cells. We already know that without oxygen inside the cells we cannot create the energy we need to move our metabolism.

Therefore, when a person suffers or has problems with their thyroid gland they begin to suffer from slow metabolism. The malfunctioning of the thyroid is known as **hypothyroidism**. Hypothyroidism is a condition in which the thyroid gland produces an insufficient amount of the hormones that control metabolism, the temperature, and the energy of the body. This condition is characterized by symptoms such as depression, hair loss, cold extremities, constipation, dry skin, difficulty slimming down, continuous fatigue, digestive problems, and continuous infections.

The thyroid gland produces a hormone called T4. It is so named because it has four atoms of the iodine mineral . This T4 hormone is not an active hormone but a storage hormone. Through the action of an enzyme [87] called deiodinase, the body converts the T4 hormone into the T3 hormone and it is so called because after the transformation, it has three atoms of iodine, instead of the four it originally had.

The T3 hormone is an active hormone and is the one that regulates the oxygen entry into the cells, producing energy and increasing the body temperature. T4 hormone would be like having oil and T3 would be like having gasoline, which is the active and usable product of oil.

There is another very important hormone called TSH (Thyroid Stimulating Hormone). This is a messenger hormone that the brain segregates to command the thyroid to produce more T4, to convert it into T3 and keep the body's metabolism and temperature functioning. When the brain detects low T3 hormone activity in the

---

[87] enzyme: enzymes are proteins that participate in achieving changes and transformations of other substances. For example, there is an enzyme that transforms cholesterol and converts it into the estrogen hormone. There are different enzymes that are used to digest fats, proteins, and carbohydrates. There are enzymes involved in all processes in the body.

cells it then produces more TSH hormone to stimulate the thyroid gland to produce more T4 hormone that can then be converted to T3. It is a system where the brain constantly monitors the amounts of T3 available and orders the thyroid gland to produce more T4 through its production of TSH.

This system is the METABOLISM COMMAND CONTROL CENTER. Know that keeping your thyroid gland functioning properly will help you to be healthy and have a truly optimal metabolism. However, this gland is very delicate and can be damaged very easily. As we saw, the consumption of enemy substances such as soy and other foods with high amounts of goitrogens such as peanuts, cassava and cabbage can harm it. In addition to these foods, sadly I must tell you that bread also harms you.

I know this may be bad news for you, but what happens with bread, besides the fact that it is very high in refined carbohydrates, is that in its manufacturing process a mineral called bromide (potassium bromate) is added to it, with the intention of giving the bread that fluffy and soft consistency that we like so much. Without the bromide, the consistency of the bread is a hard and dry one. The main problem with bromide is that it is composed almost the same as the mineral iodine, of which thyroid hormones are composed. So, when the thyroid is producing these hormones, it uses bromide instead of the mineral iodine. This results in super deficient T4 and T3 hormones that do not do their job as they should.

Originally, iodine was added to bread to give it its softness, but iodine became very scarce and expensive, which is why manufacturers replaced it with bromide without knowing the damage it would cause to our metabolism. So, if you are a lover of bread, pizza and other products based on wheat flour you should be careful because they may contain bromide and, besides affecting your thyroid, it has also been associated with depression and cancer, which is why its use has been banned in many countries, except in the United States and several Latin American countries.

Other substances that affect the functioning of the thyroid gland are pesticides, mercury, and fluoride. Mercury is known to be a highly toxic metal that also competes with and displaces iodine from the body's cells. Only a little bit does harm, however, amalgams used in dental work contain mercury. On the other hand, fluoride was used to slow down the thyroid in people suffering from hyperthyroidism. It literally slows down the functioning of the thyroid gland, but in many countries, fluoride is added to the drinking water that comes into homes and most toothpastes contain it as well.

Something that is extremely harmful to the functioning of the thyroid gland is the excessive consumption of Type F Foods (refined carbohydrates, starches). Note that most people with obesity or overweight also have hypothyroidism and this is only those who have been diagnosed with it.

There are thousands of people who have problems with the functioning of their thyroid gland but have not been given a medical diagnosis of hypothyroidism because it is not reflected in their lab test results. The reality is that, if the person suffers from several of the manifestations we will see below, they have hypothyroidism which we call subclinical hypothyroidism[88].

The most common symptoms felt by people who have problems with their thyroid gland are the following:

☐ high cholesterol
☐ hair loss when combing
☐ continuous tiredness
☐ depression
☐ difficulty slimming down
☐ constipation
☐ cold extremities

☐ recurrent infections
☐ insomnia
☐ loss of interest in sex
☐ memory loss
☐ digestive problems
☐ dry skin
☐ fluid retention

If you experience one or more of these symptoms, you are probably having problems with your thyroid gland and with your metabolism and overall health. The thyroid performs several very important functions such as:

---

[88] subclinical hypothyroidism: a type of hypothyroidism that many people have that is not detected by thyroid laboratory tests that measure hormones (TSH, T4, T3). This type of subclinical hypothyroidism is very prevalent among people with obesity who suffer from slow metabolism. There are leading physicians who recognize and treat it. There are other doctors who do not give it any credit and prefer to medicate their patient with an antidepressant that creates more obesity and uncontrolled diabetes anyway.

1. **Absorbs the iodine contained in food.**
   In fact, thyroid cells are the only cells that absorb iodine efficiently.

2. It takes the iodine from food and converts it into the T4 hormones (it has four atoms of iodine) and T3 (it has three atoms of iodine).

3. **Regulates body processes and body temperature.**
   The T4 and T3 hormones produced by the thyroid regulate the speed of all body processes and body temperature. In that sense the thyroid would be equivalent to the accelerator pedal of your car and to the thermostat (temperature regulator) of an air conditioner.

4. **Energy creation and regulation of metabolic rate.**
   The thyroid regulates the rate at which the body's cells burn or use nutrients to produce energy.

5. **Reduces cholesterol.**
   If the thyroid improves, cholesterol is reduced, and if it worsens, cholesterol increases. One of the causes of high cholesterol is having hypothyroidism.

6. **Regulates storage and fat burning.**
   From the thyroid the body's ability is controlled, both to break down and use stored fats, as well as to create and store new fat, as it happens with obesity.

7. **Increases oxygen utilization.**
   When hypothyroidism is present, the person experiences fatigue or weakness due to lack of oxygen in the cells.

For these reasons, when the thyroid does not function properly, as it does among people who consume refined carbohydrates in excess, ALL the body's functions are affected.

The good news is that the opposite is also true. When a person works to restore their metabolism, not only do they slim down, but their thyroid function is also improved. Approximately 50% of the people who receive our help to restore the metabolism at NaturalSlim have thyroid problems. The problems of hypothyroidism and obesity are closely related.

If you suspect you are suffering from sub-clinical hypothyroidism, the only way to detect if you have it is to take your body temperature. The thyroid oversees the regulation of BODY TEMPERATURE. It is as if it were the thermostat (temperature regulator) of your body. The human body, to be healthy, must operate very close to NORMAL temperature which is 37 degrees Celsius or 98.6 degrees Fahrenheit.

When your body temperature is a little higher than normal (37° C or 98.6° F) it is called a fever. If this happens, we go to the doctor right away. Curiously, when our temperature becomes quite cold, NO ONE SAYS ANYTHING

AND IT IS IGNORED. Well, both hypothyroidism and the slow metabolism and emotional depression, or lack of energy that often accompanies them, only occur when the body temperature, due to hypothyroid problems, is reduced below the critical point (36.5° C or 97.8° F).

When your body generates little heat and becomes cold, what it means is that your thyroid is too deficient, so oxygen is lacking in the cells and your body cools down, just as if it were a fire going out to turn into ashes. If you do identify with several of the symptoms of subclinical hypothyroidism, but have been told you do not have a thyroid problem, and are curious to know the truth, TAKE YOUR BODY TEMPERATURE.

The most accurate thermometers are glass thermometers, but unfortunately, they are no longer produced. So, when purchasing a digital thermometer be sure to buy the one that takes the temperature the most slowly. You will see that in stores, they market thermometers that they say they are very fast. But for the temperature to be as accurate as possible <u>you should buy the digital thermometer that does the process more slowly</u> and you will get a more accurate result.

STEPS TO TAKE A TEMPERATURE AND IDENTIFY SUBCLINICAL HYPOTHYROIDISM

1. You should take your temperature before eating.

2. The temperature should be taken three times a day. If you have a glass thermometer, you should leave the thermometer under the tongue for three to four minutes. If it is a digital thermometer, remember to choose the one that calculates the temperature the slowest so that it is more accurate.

3. After taking your temperature before each meal, write it down.

4. At the end of the day, the three temperatures should be added together and then averaged.

5. You must do this process for three consecutive days to observe if you have subclinical hypothyroidism.

| Example Using a Fahrenheit Degree System ||||
meal	temperature	sum	daily average is
breakfast	96.5°	96.5°	288.9
lunch	95.4°	+ 95.4°	------- = 96.3° F
dinner	97°	+ 97°	3

Example Using a Celsius Degree System			
meal	temperature	sum	daily average is
breakfast	35°	35°	106.5
lunch	35.5°	+ 35.5°	------- = 35.5° C
dinner	36°	+ 36°	3

Another factor that greatly affects the thyroid is stress. In fact, stress is what affects this gland the most. Most women who are having problems with their thyroid today started having problems with their thyroid right after some emotionally traumatic or painful event. For example, after a contentious divorce, or after a painful and stressful childbirth, even after a car accident or after the loss of a loved one. Likewise, if you suffer from internal stress in the body due to a health condition or for an unbalanced nervous system, it will also affect your thyroid.

On the other hand, the thyroid has specific needs of some nutrients, vitamins and minerals that, if they are not covered and there is a deficiency of any of these necessary elements, cause it to fail in its function. To function properly the thyroid cannot be deficient in any of the following substances, vitamins, and minerals: iodine, zinc, magnesium, copper, manganese, selenium, and the amino acid L-Tyrosine. If any of these are missing, your thyroid will not be able to produce efficient hormones to keep your metabolism functioning optimally.

In conclusion, we must take care of our thyroid gland, which together with the brain and the nervous system, are the CONTROL CENTER OF OUR METABOLISM. We must manage stress and calm our nervous system, have the correct nutrition in proportion to the 3x1 Diet so that we do not consume an excess of refined carbohydrates and avoid the consumption of the substances that do so much damage to it. This will ensure that we restore our metabolism and improve our health.

Pathway to an Ultra-Powerful Metabolism

👀 **The thyroid gland, together with the brain, make up the control center of our metabolism.**
- The hormones produced by the thyroid regulate how much oxygen can enter the cells for energy production.
- If the thyroid gland becomes affected, it produces inefficient hormones and the necessary oxygen does not reach the cells, so less energy is produced than we need, and the metabolism shuts down.
- We must help our thyroid gland by doing the following:
  - handling the internal and external stress levels of the body
  - avoiding the consumption of substances that affect its functioning
  - controlling the consumption of Type F Foods (FATTENING), feeding ourselves in proportion to the 3x1 Die

- supplementing our body with the vitamins, minerals and amino acids that the thyroid needs to produce efficient hormones
- Body temperature says it all. If we suspect we have subclinical hypothyroidism we can find out by taking our body temperature.

👀 Answer the following questions

1. Write here all the hypothyroidism symptoms, presented in this chapter, that you suffer from,

2. What actions will you take to improve the functioning of your thyroid gland and your metabolism?

THE AGGRESSOR FOODS

In this book, *Ultra-Powerful Metabolism*, I want to share with you what I consider to be one of my most important discoveries for restoring metabolism and improving health. It is a discovery that we could almost say produces miracles in those who apply it. It was something I discovered when I was researching the topic of diabetes and prediabetes to write my book *Problem-Free Diabetes*.

After many, many years of experiencing the incredible improvements that people with diabetes were having by participating in the NaturalSlim program, I wondered why do people with diabetes continue to die, with amputations or blindness, if there is a natural way to avoid all the damages of diabetes? At that time, I was preparing to write a book that would explain in a very simple way how to control diabetes and its damage without the need for excessive medications.

More than twenty years ago I, Frank Suárez, was just an obese, prediabetic and sick patient. Having failed with all the "expert recommendations" given to me by doctors and nutritionists, I became an independent researcher specializing in only one subject, which finally gave me good results, and for which it became my passion: metabolism. I realized that issuing opinions on how to control diabetes, without being a doctor, would easily bring me accusations from the medical class that might resent my meddling in a disease like diabetes that only doctors control.

Since the topic of diabetes control is one that forcefully requires the expert attention of a physician, I took on the task of making sure that each of my recommendations to the diabetic patient or the person caring for that diabetic patient was supported by science. I did not want the diabetic patients or physicians reading *Problem-Free Diabetes* to think that my book was based on my opinions, so I ended up documenting my diabetes book with over eight hundred references of clinical studies[89].

To further assure myself that what I would be expressing in *Problem-Free Diabetes* really worked to control diabetes without medications, I decided to recruit twenty-five medicated diabetic patients and with them do a medically supervised clinical study at NaturalSlim to scientifically measure the results of my recommendations. The study with the twenty-five diabetics lasted thirteen weeks and we were able to prove and demonstrate, under medical supervision, that in fact the method I had created to restore metabolism produced impressive results in diabetic patients, as evidenced by laboratory tests.

---

[89] clinical studies: clinical studies are publications of scientific studies that have been carried out by physicians and scientific researchers from universities and gather scientific evidence on a subject related to medicine or health.

Among the twenty-five diabetic patients who participated, we observed how seven of the eleven who were using injected insulin had to be completely removed from insulin by their physicians because they no longer needed it. For the other four who still needed to use insulin, their doctors had to reduce their daily doses to only one-third or less of the dose they were using at the start of the study. In addition to slimming down, it turned out that twenty-one of the twenty-five diabetic patients reported reductions in their medication doses that were ordered by their own physicians, including other diabetes medications plus thyroid and hypertension medications. Finally, this clinical study conducted at NaturalSlim was published in scientific magazines by medical researchers from the Medical Sciences Campus of the University of Puerto Rico, under the title METABOLIC CORRECTION AS A TOOL TO IMPROVE TYPE 2 DIABETES MANAGEMENT.

I have told you about this journey of my research into the mysteries of the body's metabolism to introduce you to the subject of AGGRESSOR FOODS, and to give you the opportunity for you to understand how I made this discovery, which you can use to your advantage to achieve an Ultra-Powerful Metabolism. I am careful never to exaggerate in my opinions concerning metabolism issues. But I consider that the discovery of the AGGRESSOR FOODS is so important that I can tell you, with all certainty, the following assertion:

By learning to detect and then remove AGGRESSOR FOODS from your diet, <u>which are different for everyone,</u>

you will have the opportunity to solve health problems that no other way, treatment, or medications could solve.

Let me explain what AGGRESSOR FOODS (AF) are and how I discovered them. While we were doing the medically supervised clinical study with the twenty-five diabetic patients who visited our NaturalSlim facilities in Puerto Rico on a weekly basis, we saw how each week the study participants continued to slim down and each time they needed less and less prescription medications.

The purpose of the clinical study with NaturalSlim diabetic patients was to demonstrate that when Type F (FATTENING) foods were reduced with the help of the 3x1 Diet and good hydration, diabetes could be reversed and many of the diabetic medications would become unnecessary. This was the same thing we had experienced with diabetic patients participating in the NaturalSlim program, but this time we wanted to demonstrate it with laboratory evidence and under medical supervision.

During the study, week after week, we were seeing pure MIRACLES among the twenty-five participating diabetic patients: fewer medications, elimination of insulin, impotent diabetic men who had regained sexual potency, recovery of sight in some who were losing it, and other health improvements that could be considered miracles.

The physician we hired to oversee the study, Dr. Fernando Álvarez, was impressed with the results because, in his medical practice of over twenty years, he had never seen diabetics improve so much or so fast just by restoring metabolism.

The results of impressive improvements we were experiencing week after week with these twenty-five diabetics using simple techniques of reducing Type F Foods and good hydration to reduce glucose levels, proved to me what I already suspected: <u>There is truly no intention by medical or pharmaceutical organizations to prevent the deaths and damage of diabetes without medications</u>. **Sick people are a good business**, and it becomes obvious that if patients are cured or controlled without medications it would destroy the medical and pharmaceutical empire.

With this clinical study we wanted to demonstrate and document the evidence of how much health improvement could be achieved by improving metabolism and we were accomplishing it. Since the main problem in both diabetes and obesity are the EXCESSIVELY HIGH LEVELS OF GLUCOSE, we asked the twenty-five diabetics in the study to report their glucose (blood sugar) levels to us on a weekly basis.

Glucose levels are measured with the help of a glucometer, which is a measuring instrument used by diabetic patients to accurately measure blood glucose levels.

I was able to observe that some diabetics were able to reduce their glucose levels to a totally normal (non-diabetic) level by simply eliminating rice, which is an essential part of the typical Puerto Rican diet. I observed that other diabetics could stop using insulin when they stopped eating bread, crackers or wheat flour.

For example, one of the twenty-five diabetics patients in the study had needed daily insulin injections for more than ten years. When he stopped eating rice, his glucose levels returned to normal (non-diabetic). For some reason the RICE was triggering his glucose to sky-high levels and that was what was forcing him to use insulin. After he stopped eating rice, he used to eat every day, his glucose measurements normalized (normal non-diabetic levels) and his doctor ordered him to eliminate insulin completely. For this patient, RICE was what I later called an AGGRESSOR FOOD.

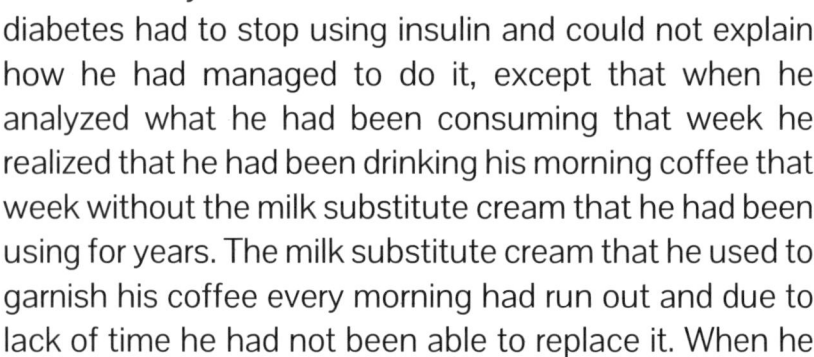

Another participant in the clinical study for the control of diabetes had to stop using insulin and could not explain how he had managed to do it, except that when he analyzed what he had been consuming that week he realized that he had been drinking his morning coffee that week without the milk substitute cream that he had been using for years. The milk substitute cream that he used to garnish his coffee every morning had run out and due to lack of time he had not been able to replace it. When he told me this, I went to investigate what ingredients were used to manufacture this milk substitute creamer and I observed that its main ingredient was CORN (corn solids).

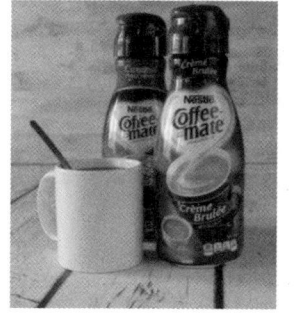

I asked him to try drinking his coffee again with that milk substitute creamer and when he did so, he was horrified because his glucose levels rose to diabetic levels and again he would need insulin to reduce it.

I did more tests with this patient, who kindly volunteered to help me research this issue, and we discovered that any product containing CORN would spike his glucose. His body's reaction to CORN was so violent that any food whose ingredients contained CORN would throw his glucose out of control for up to several days. He had discovered that CORN in all its forms was an AGGRESSOR FOOD for his body.

So, I continued to research the topic of AGGRESSOR FOODS with hundreds of people (diabetics and non-diabetics) who learned to use a glucometer to detect and remove those foods that aggravate them. Whenever the human body is affected by stress, glucose is triggered to a much higher level in response to stress. We know that stress is fattening, and we also know that it is fattening simply because as glucose levels rise, the body converts that glucose into fat for storage.

AGGRESSOR FOODS are foods that cause STRESS to the body causing a reaction of the Excited Nervous System (see chapter WE ARE ALL NOT THE SAME) and in turn that forces the body to prepare itself to "fight or flee", which increases glucose in the blood.

AGGRESSOR FOODS are foods that your body, for hereditary reasons, violently rejects, so consuming them causes your body a type of allergic reaction that causes severe stress to the nervous system. As you already know stress is fattening, since any kind of stress always impacts your body's nervous system and will always result in HIGH GLUCOSE.

HIGH GLUCOSE is the common factor between obesity and diabetes. In addition, it can easily be the cause of cancer, hypothyroidism, depression, insomnia, blindness, kidney damage, heart attacks and many other health conditions.

I discovered that each person, because of genetic differences, has different AGGRESSOR FOODS. What an AF is for me is not an AF for my wife, nor does it have to be for you. Even within the same family, some children's aggressor is corn while it is wheat to others; mom's aggressor is coffee, and dad are almonds and tomatoes.

In my case, rice, wheat, pork, chocolate, coffee (that is why I drink green tea), and dairy products (cheeses, butter that comes from cow milk) are aggressors to me. Corn, wheat, and shrimps are my wife Elizabeth's aggressors. In my 89-year-old mother Irma's case, her aggressor foods are rice, beans, and wheat. So in my family we are all different, and we all have different AGGRESSOR FOODS.

The biggest mistake that can exist on this subject is to think that there can be any food that is "so healthy" that it cannot be an AGGRESSOR FOOD for you. The only way I have discovered so far to detect AGGRESSOR FOODS is with the help of a GLUCOMETER. That is why I recorded several videos on my MetabolismoTV YouTube channel where I explain in detail how to detect your AGGRESSOR FOODS. After detecting the AGGRESSOR FOODS and removing them we have seen dramatic improvements such as these five cases:

1. A 24-year-old man from Puerto Rico, who suffered from psychotic attacks, discovered that his psychotic attacks, which caused him to be hospitalized for weeks in a psychiatric hospital, were caused by eating rice. He stopped eating rice when he discovered with his glucometer that it triggered his glucose, and his psychosis went away. Months later he decided to try just a little rice and ended up in the psychiatric hospital again. He finally realized that RICE is a violent Aggressor Food for him.

2. A very thin Mexican track and field runner lived in frustration because, although she ran ten kilometers a day, she had never been able to eliminate her abdominal fat (belly), which was visibly prominent. The belly disappeared in less

than two weeks after she discovered that her main Aggressor Food was CORN and stopped consuming it.

3. A young woman from Costa Rica, had a cancerous tumor in her uterus. Upon discovering that WHEAT (bread, cookies, flour, gluten) was her AGGRESSOR FOOD, she stopped consuming it and automatically the tumor began to shrink, to the point that her oncologist (cancer specialist) discharged her.

4. A very thin man from Mexico had very high blood pressure even with medications and feared he might have a heart attack at any moment. He tested with his glucometer all the foods he was accustomed to eating. Finally, he discovered that his Aggressor Food was TOMATO. He began to avoid tomato, and his blood pressure normalized to such a point within two months, that his doctor first reduced and then took him off the high blood pressure medications.

5. A young man from Colombia suffered from anxiety attacks that made him imagine he was being persecuted. This young man was about to lose his job when he watched one of my videos about Aggressor Foods on my video channel, MetabolismoTV. He bought a glucometer, watched the videos where I explain how to detect Aggressor Foods and discovered that he had

several Aggressor Foods like corn and wheat. But the most violent Aggressor Food that triggered his anxiety attacks was COFFEE and CAFFEINE. He knew his Aggressor Food was caffeine because the anxiety attack would hit him if he drank a cup of coffee or if he drank a Coke which also contains caffeine.

From what I have observed, rare is the person who does not have some AGGRESSOR FOOD that they are consuming without realizing that it is causing destruction to their body. When glucose (blood sugar) exceeds 130 mg/dl (milligrams per deciliter) the cells suffer sometimes irreparable damage (see the book *Problem-Free Diabetes*).

The three foods we have discovered that seem to be the most common AGGRESSOR FOODS in the population are what we at NaturalSlim call the "WRC". The WRC comes from joining the first letters of Wheat, Rice and Corn. However, we have seen in the practice of NaturalSlim centers that AGGRESSOR FOODS can be foods as varied as: chicken, turkey, pork, beef, shrimp, eggs, tomatoes, cucumbers, lettuce, carrots, onions, peppers, strawberries, apples, oranges, peaches, grapes, potatoes, sweet potatoes, corn, wheat, beans, peppers, chocolate, almonds, soy and dairy (cheese, yogurt, butter), among many others. Each person is different and therefore not all of us are affected by the same types of foods.

Consuming AGGRESSOR FOODS causes severe stress to the body's nervous system, thus bringing glucose levels to an abnormally high range (over 130 mg/dl). In practice with thousands of people throughout the nine countries where NaturalSlim operates, we observed that consuming some AGGRESSOR FOODS or several of them can be the cause of all these manifestations, which easily disappear once we detect them and remove them from our diet:

- anxiety attacks, depression
- mustache or beard in women
- candidiasis – candida yeast
- headaches, migraines
- back pain
- constipation
- lack of energy
- abdominal fat
- hypothyroidism with nodules
- bad sleep quality
- hands and cold feet
- irregular menstruation
- digestive problems
- hair falls when combing your hair

HEALTH-DESTROYING GLUCOSE SPIKES

Why do diabetic patients have to have their legs amputated? Why is there so much blindness among people with diabetes? Why do diabetic patients have kidney damage? Why do people with diabetes have five times more cancer than people without diabetes?

The answer to all the above questions about what causes amputations, blindness, kidney damage and cancer in diabetic patients is only one:

Excessively high glucose levels (more than 130 mg/dl) that cause the death of body cells.

You should know that OBESITY and DIABETES have a common cause: **excessively high glucose levels.**

It is impossible to become fat or obese if you do not first raise your glucose to very high levels. It is also impossible to be diagnosed by your doctor as a diabetic if you do not first raise and maintain your glucose at very high levels. The same EXCESS GLUCOSE that causes OBESITY is the same EXCESS GLUCOSE that, when kept high all the time, doctors call DIABETES.

What makes the human body fat and destroys it is EXCESSIVELY HIGH LEVELS OF GLUCOSE. What feeds a cancerous tumor is EXCESSIVELY HIGH LEVELS OF GLUCOSE. Glucose spikes above 130 mg/dl (destructive glucose level) caused by AGGRESSOR FOODS you are unknowingly consuming can take their toll.

Even if you have not been diagnosed with diabetes you should know that, if you are unknowingly consuming AGGRESSOR FOODS, you may find out too late if you allow time to pass and the damage continues to accumulate, eventually developing into diabetes, arthritis, or cancer.

As far as I know, there is no previous explanation as to how a food that we consider "healthy" can cause an abnormal rise in glucose (blood sugar) to health-destroying levels. I guarantee you that it IS TRUE that AGGRESSOR FOODS exist and that they can gradually destroy your health. You do not have to believe me. You can prove it yourself with the help of a glucometer. The glucometer does not lie!

Any food that causes a stress reaction to your body's nervous system and raises your blood glucose above 130 mg/dl will gradually DESTROY YOUR HEALTH!

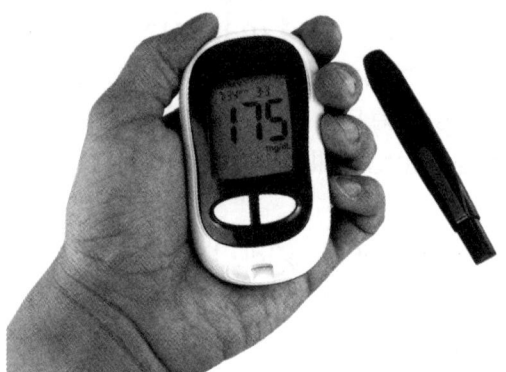

GLUCOSE ABOVE 130 MG/DL IS DESTRUCTIVE

You do not have to be diabetic to obtain a glucometer, learn how to use it and learn to detect your own AGGRESSOR FOODS.

When purchasing a glucometer, you should try to buy the glucometer that uses the least expensive test strips. The glucometer business is like the printer business, where they will almost give you the printer for free if you are tied to their brand of ink cartridge.

The glucometer manufacturers almost give you the glucometer meter for free and then charge you for the expensive strips. The manufacturer makes the most money on the strips, not on the glucometer. I have seen discount stores like Wal-Mart bring to market glucometers that are inexpensive and for which you can get very inexpensive strips.

THE RULES FOR FINDING AGGRESSOR FOODS

1. THE MAIN MISTAKE is to think that there may be some food or drink that may not be an aggressor food for your body. You must be suspicious of EVERYTHING to be successful!

2. So far, the best way to find an aggressor food is to take your glucometer measurement before eating and two hours after eating, as explained in my videos on MetabolismoTV.

3. Research reflects that true Aggressor Foods tend to be OBVIOUS because they produce large glucose surges that can be noticed within two hours.

4. Look for OBVIOUS glucose rises. Example: before eating your glucose was 80 mg/dl and two hours later it was still 110-120 mg/dl. Example: before eating you were at 90mg/dl, you consumed rice and two hours later you were at 120-130 mg/dl.

5. An Aggressor Food can both RAISE your blood glucose too high and LOWER your blood glucose too low. There are some Aggressor Foods that can stress your body so much that they force it to produce excess of insulin, thus abnormally lowering glucose within two hours.

6. Never classify a food as an aggressor food unless you check it again with another measurement from your glucometer. If it is a true aggressor food, it will attack you again and so you can check it.

7. Allow your body to recover and normalize after the aggression caused by an aggressor food. Wait for your glucose to stabilize in its normal range before testing out new Aggressor Foods again. Some Aggressor Foods are so strong that they can destabilize your glucose for up to twenty-four hours, as we have seen happen in some cases with corn and the products derived from corn. This may be the aggressor effect of genetically modified corn.

8. Take and record the measurement of your GLUCOSE AT FASTING (upon waking-up) every day and keep a record of the measurements. You will see that your glucose at fasting will get lower and lower each day as you remove your Aggressor Foods from your diet. If you do not have diabetes and your glucose at fasting is over 85 mg/dl, you

are almost certainly consuming one or more Aggressor Foods.

I wish you success in your hunt for AGGRESSOR FOODS! Finding and removing them can save your life or greatly improve your health. Accomplishing this requires discipline and takes work, but the results are sure to pleasantly surprise you.

To learn how to locate your AGGRESSOR FOODS, including tricks to puncture yourself to extract a drop of blood without pain, I recommend you watch the following videos from my MetabolismoTV channel on YouTube:

Free Educational Videos MetabolismoTV

- Episode # 705: Detecting Aggressor Foods
- Episode # 720: Exposing Three Aggressor Foods
- Episode # 696: The Aggressor Foods
- Episode # 697: The Aggressor Foods, Part 2
- Episode # 942: The Aggressor Foods Always Give a Warning

There are some people who are afraid of puncturing (pricking) themselves and prefer not to make the effort to know exactly how their body is reacting to the different foods they eat. In other words, they prefer not to even know so long as they do not have to prick themselves. This is a form of slow suicide. It is like the phrase "what you don't know, can't hurt you" that only reflects an inability to confront a problem or threat. However, it is up to me to tell you the TRUTH because if I do not, I will harm those who do care to know the truth and who are willing to confront life's challenges. In my practice of more than twenty years in the NaturalSlim centers I have helped hundreds of thousands of people to recover their health, to eliminate their dependence on medications and in some cases, they even managed to stop cancer.

To find my own body's AGGRESSOR FOODS, I bought an inexpensive glucometer with 200 of the cheapest test strips I could find and set out to test ALL the different foods I ate for a period of about 30 days. I opened a small file of notes on my mobile phone and made notes of everything I ate. I measured each of the foods before and two hours after eating them. I gradually discovered that most foods did not aggravate me. But I was also able to detect and check with my glucometer which are my AGGRESSOR FOODS. My wife did the same, as did my 89-year-old mother, who today is in such good health that her family doctor simply cannot believe such health in a woman of her age.

From my perspective there is no body or health situation that cannot be improved or controlled with the help of the knowledge about the metabolism. The issue of AGGRESSOR FOODS is a FACT, whether you dare confront it or not. I have seen several miracles, healing, and recoveries in abundance after the full exercise of detecting and removing what may be the AGGRESSOR FOODS from your body. The enemy of your health is hidden inside your body. With the help of a glucometer and being very patient and disciplined, the hidden enemy can be unmasked and thus add long years of healthy and vibrant life.

Pathway to an Ultra-Powerful Metabolism

ᅗ The Consumption of Aggressor Foods maintains high levels of glucose in the blood, which damages your metabolism.
- Having high blood glucose levels cause the body to create more fat and will not allow you to slim down.
- Also, having blood glucose levels above the danger point (130 mg/dl) causes diabetes and even cancer.
- The most common Aggressor Foods among most people are Wheat, Rice and Corn.
- AGGRESSOR FOODS are not necessarily all Type F Foods. Everyone is different and foods such as meats may also be aggressors to your body.
- Discovering and eliminating Aggressor Foods from your diet will prevent excessively high blood glucose levels, internal body stress and help restore your metabolism.

ᅗ Answer the following questions
1. Make a list of the foods that you suspect may be causing an aggression to your body. What noticeable reactions do they cause in your body when you eat them?

2. What actions will you take now that you know the truth about Aggressor Foods?

THE HORMONAL BALANCE

All organs, glands, tissues, muscles, nerves and bones in the body are influenced by hormones. Hormones in turn are very powerful substances that can give orders to the body cells and can therefore modify the structure of the body.

Our body produces countless hormones to carry messages through all its systems. But there are several very important hormones among which there must be a balance to ensure the proper functioning of our body and our metabolism.

Women's and men's bodies produce two hormones called estrogen and testosterone. The balance between the amount of these in each body will set the traits that differentiate female bodies from male bodies. For example, the female estrogen hormone communicates messages to the body's cells that create feminine features: breasts, no beard, more fat and less muscle; while the male testosterone hormone carries the opposite message of creating male bodies: no breasts, beard, less fat and more muscle.

A woman's body is always more complex than a man's precisely because of her hormonal system. It is a known fact that men slim down easily, but women have a much harder time slimming down. This is due to several reasons such as the following:

- A man's body has more musculature and therefore consumes more energy and burns fat more easily.
- A man's body produces a lot of the male testosterone hormone which is a muscle building and fat burning hormone. A woman's body produces a lot of estrogen hormone which is a hormone that stores fat in the body.
- Women tend to have higher emotional stress levels than men and therefore produce higher levels of the stress hormone cortisol, which is a hormone that accumulates fat in the abdomen and hips.

For these reasons, women always slim down slower than men. One of the reasons, excess estrogen hormone, has to do with a condition that many women suffer from, especially when they are overweight. The condition is called ESTROGEN PREDOMINANCE.

The estrogen hormone is a group of several substances that are vital in a woman's body. Without estrogen, there would be no pregnancy, nor would there be smooth female skin, nor menstruation, nor breasts in a woman. A woman's body balances estrogen with another hormone produced during ovulation called progesterone.

Progesterone is the hormone that, as its name reflects, allows for gestation or getting pregnant. A woman's body depends on a certain hormonal balance between these two hormones, estrogen and progesterone.

It is well known that estrogen is produced in the ovaries of women, but few people know that body fat also produces estrogen with the help of an enzyme called aromatase. Fat produces estrogen and is the reason why very obese men develop breasts and become feminized even in their tone of voice. ESTROGEN PREDOMINANCE is a condition where the body continues to produce estrogen from stored fat.

In women's bodies, estrogen continues to be produced from fat even when the ovaries are not functioning. When estrogen is not being balanced in the body by progesterone, which is only produced during ovulation, estrogen dominates the body's internal environment, continues to accumulate more fat, and does not allow women to slim down.

That is precisely the problem with the estrogen hormone, that it accumulates fat and causes fattening. This is a well-known fact since a few years ago pig and chicken breeders tried to increase the weight of their animals by supplementing their diet with estrogen to fatten them up. This was on the front pages of the country as a scandal and as a result many people decided not to continue consuming chicken meat. As far as I understand, this practice is no longer carried out, but many people were shocked and refused to eat chicken for fear that it contains estrogen.

The predominance of estrogen in women can cause manifestations such as the following:

- ☐ fat accumulation on the hips and abdomen
- ☐ recurrent candidiasis (resistant yeast infections)
- ☐ autoimmune conditions such as: lupus, multiple sclerosis, fibromyalgia
- ☐ difficulty or slowness in slimming down
- ☐ difficulty conceiving
- ☐ edema (water accumulation)
- ☐ lack of energy or continuous fatigue
- ☐ history of breast or uterine cancer
- ☐ history of fibroids, adenomas, or vaginal polyps
- ☐ history of having natural miscarriages
- ☐ painful menstruation or cramps
- ☐ osteoporosis (bone loss)
- ☐ facial hair
- ☐ loss of libido (sexual interest or appetite)
- ☐ menstrual blood in excess
- ☐ breast tenderness
- ☐ too light sleep or difficulty sleeping

To maintain a balance between the amount of the estrogen hormone and the amount of the progesterone hormone in women's bodies, I recommend that women use a natural progesterone cream. Natural progesterone not only maintains a balance of estrogen in the body but also has the following qualities:

- helps to sleep deeper and to have a restful sleep
- helps to recover bone lost due to osteoporosis

- helps reduce fat in the abdomen and hips
- increases a woman's libido (interest in sex)
- has an anti-aging effect on the body
- has a calming and antidepressant effect

The cream should be used only for twenty-one consecutive days in a month, to prevent the body from getting used to it and stop having an effect, besides we want to create a cycle as if the body itself was producing it through ovulation. If the woman is still menstruating, she should start using the progesterone cream on the first day of bleeding of her menstrual period, for twenty-one days, stop using it on the twenty-first day, and then start using it again when the first day of bleeding of her next menstruation period begins. If the woman is no longer menstruating, I recommend that she start using it on the first day of the calendar month until the twenty-first day and then rest for seven days, until the first day of the next month.

This cream is available in natural health centers and can even be purchased on the Internet. For women who have experienced a lot of difficulty in losing weight and especially for those who have accumulated a lot of fat on their hips and abdomen (caused by estrogen) natural progesterone cream is an excellent help.

Also, a women's ovaries produce some testosterone naturally. As we already know, the testosterone hormone is the male hormone. When there is an imbalance between the amount of testosterone and estrogen in the body you can see that a woman starts to grow a mustache and a beard.

This unbalance in the correct amount of testosterone occurs because there is a problem in the liver. One of the functions of the liver is that it reprocesses and detoxifies the body of any substances it does not need. The liver also produces a substance called hormone binding globulin. The hormone binding globulin is called globulin because it is like a globe. Under normal conditions, the liver finds the testosterone produced by the ovaries and since the woman's body does not need it, it covers it with the globulin (puts it like the inside of a globe) and converts the testosterone into an inactive hormone in the woman's body and thus the body can eliminate it.

When we see a woman that is growing a lot of beard and mustache it means that her liver is not able to produce the globulin to inactivate the testosterone produced by her ovaries. So, the testosterone is staying free and active. The main reason that has been discovered that is not allowing the liver to produce globulin is that there is too much insulin hormone in the body.

The insulin hormone gives the message to the liver not to produce globulin. As we already know, the EXCESS OF INSULIN in the body is produced by the excessive amount of consumption of Type F Foods (refined carbohydrates, fattening). So, the solution is to restore the metabolism, reduce the excess consumption of refined carbohydrates and slim down to lower the amount of insulin in the body that prevents the liver from making the globulin that inactivates testosterone in women's bodies. You can see more information on this topic in Episode #1342 of MetabolismoTV.

However, hormonal balance is also vital in men. Testosterone hormone deficiency in men causes them to lose muscle mass, accumulate fat, their bodies become flabby, and their sexual potency is affected.

The testosterone hormone is named so because it is produced in the testicles of men, but it is also produced in the ovaries of women and in the adrenal glands of both men and women. Testosterone is responsible for the creation of the eggs and sperm in men. Testosterone is also involved in the functioning of the immune system and in wound healing. In addition, testosterone controls sexual desire.

A man's body produces a lot of testosterones. In fact, it produces eight to ten times more testosterone than women, which also explains why men generally have a higher sex drive than women. Men who have healthy testosterone levels have a lower risk of heart attacks.

It is known that the testosterone hormone is the one that creates strong muscles and contributes to having a well-defined body. For this reason, when men are getting older, their bodies start to become flabbier, with less muscle and more fat. Testosterone is a hormone that, when building large and strong muscles in a man's body, also contributes to reducing body fat since, of the body's tissues, muscles are the ones that consume more fat. When a man does resistance exercises such as weightlifting, his body builds muscle, and this creates an increase in muscle mass. The muscles in turn consume body fat and create a lean, well-defined body.

If a man manages to increase his natural testosterone production, he will also achieve a substantial increase in his muscle mass and a reduction in body fat. With increased testosterone production, a man may not lose weight because the new muscles weigh two and a half times more than fat, but his body will become leaner every day and he will have energy to spare.

For more than thirty years, low-fat diets have been promoted as a way to reduce the fat content of the diet. However, since fat intake has been lowered, there has been a noticeable decrease in the production of the testosterone hormone in men's bodies and more obesity among them. The problem is that the raw building material for all hormones in the body is cholesterol; cholesterol comes from saturated fats.

Testosterone needs materials to build itself and one of them is the cholesterol from saturated fats. But by lowering your saturated fat intake, you are not able to produce the right amount of testosterone. If a person cuts down the saturated fat, it lowers cholesterol, so it lowers testosterone production.

I recommend consuming saturated fats from good meats, from grass-fed animals, good quality butter and coconut oil. In addition, the body needs zinc, which is found in oysters, egg yolks, cheeses, red meat, among other foods, and magnesium to produce healthy amounts of testosterone in both men and women. Remember that it is very important that the consumption of these foods goes according to your type of nervous system so that it does not cause additional stress to the body.

In addition to these nutritional changes, men can supplement their bodies with natural testosterone sources such as testosfen, which in clinical studies has been shown to achieve up to a 98% increase in male testosterone production. At NaturalSlim we use a formulation I developed called TESTOSTERIN, using testosfen blended with various ingredients aimed at creating a greater testosterone production and various antioxidants that are used to protect nitric oxide production in the body.

Nitric oxide is the molecule that allows men to have a satisfactory erection and was the discovery that led to the creation of erectile dysfunction medications such as Viagra. NaturalSlim male customers who use this natural supplement to increase testosterone production burn fat faster, accelerating their slim down process.

Maintaining the right levels of testosterone in a man's body will help him avoid heart problems, have more muscle and less fat, and have a better sexual performance. It is worth mentioning that men who are sexually active have a better disposition to maintain their weight and figure. When it comes to improve metabolism and slim down, a person's emotional state and general attitude towards life are determining factors. Healthy couple sex fosters a sense of affinity between the couple and is an excellent way to get rid of stress. As we know, stress produces cortisol that makes us fat, and that is why healthy sexual activity can help both men and women to slim down without so much effort.

Thus, hormonal balance in both men and women is another essential part for reaching and maintaining an Ultra-Powerful Metabolism.

Pathway to an Ultra-Powerful Metabolism

∞ **The balance between the body's hormones ensures the proper functioning of our metabolism.**
- Women should avoid estrogen dominance to truly slim down and improve their health.
- Men should maintain adequate levels of testosterone production to improve metabolism and overall health.

∞ **Answer the following questions**
1. What habits or actions have you taken in your life that have affected your body's hormonal balance?

2. What conclusions have you reached and what actions will you take after discovering the importance of the body's hormonal balance?

MOVEMENT IS LIFE

As we already know, metabolism is the sum of all the movements, actions and changes that occur in the body to convert food and nutrients into energy for survival. All the body's processes must have optimal movement for proper functioning and overall good health.

Metabolism has to do with movement. So, we want to keep our metabolism in optimal motion to be healthy. It has been proven that physical exercise increases metabolism and a sedentary lifestyle [90] decreases it. When we stop using our muscles, they get flaccid. When we use them, they grow and get stronger. The body adapts to our lifestyle.

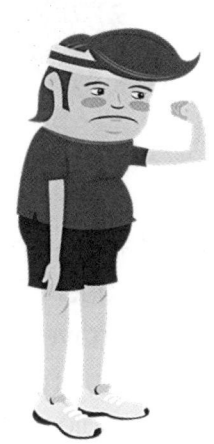

The years that I have been helping people with slow metabolism have taught me to observe what works and what does not work. Exercise is a great help and is vital to recover the maximum of your metabolism; but everything in life has its proper time and exercise is no exception to this rule. If you notice, I have not made the recommendation to exercise up to this

---

[90] sedentary life: also known as sedentarism, is the most common lifestyle. It includes little exercise and tends to increase the risk of health problems, especially obesity and cardiovascular disease. It is a frequent lifestyle in modern, highly technological cities, where everything is designed to avoid great physical effort.

point in your PATH TO AN ULTRA-POWERFUL METABOLISM and we will now see why.

Logic dictates that to exercise a person needs to expend energy, but people with a slow metabolism have very little energy! Precisely, what it means to have a slow metabolism is to have little energy because the metabolism is what produces the body's energy. People who suffer from a slow metabolism are always tired and feel weak. It is illogical to ask a weak and tired person to use what little energy they have to go to a gym to exercise. It is like going to spend money with a bank account with no funds.

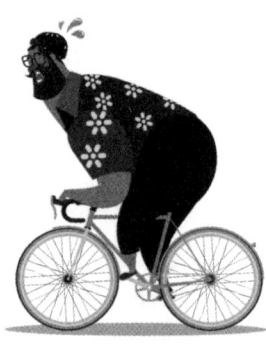

When a person with a slow metabolism, who is overweight or obese, engages in a physical exercise regimen, they are exposing themselves to failure in their attempt because they are pushing their body beyond the limit of its capabilities. Gyms have a very high percentage of members who within a few weeks of starting their exercise regimen disappear and never come back. These are weak and tired people who really do not have the necessary energy to survive the workouts for very long without collapsing from exhaustion. These are people who have a slow metabolism.

The solution to this problem is to apply the correct sequence. In life things have a sequence, they have an order. The correct sequence of actions is to improve nutrition and metabolism to obtain more energy and then invest this new energy in an exercise routine that further increases metabolism.

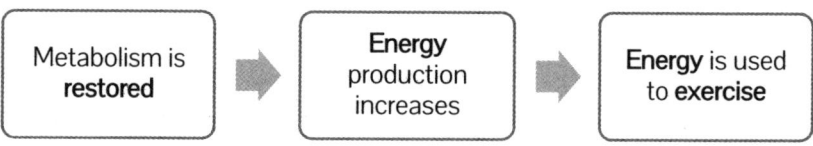

Let's look at the sequence you are already following: you already know the different factors causing you to have a slow metabolism; you are already hydrating according to your body weight; you know the difference between Type S (slimming) and Type F (fattening) foods, and you are applying your 3x1 Diet - already your metabolism and energy are improving and you can only keep improving. During this process, where you are already taking actions to improve your metabolism, you will experience an increase in your body's energy and that is the right time to start moving the body with a moderate exercise routine.

The other common cause of failure in a new exercise regimen is trying to exercise at the wrong gradient or intensity. A gradient is a level, degree, or strength of something. For example, the different temperatures of a stove are temperature gradients. In life, gradients are important. One first crawls, then walks and finally runs. They are gradients of action of different intensity and are necessary.

If a person intends to run a marathon after having spent the last twenty years of his life working in front of a computer in the office and without much energy, it is certain that he will add another failure to his list of previous failures.

The key is to start doing gentle exercise on an appropriate gradient such as walking, swimming, going to a gym, exercise based on dance routines, weightlifting or other exercise that is not stressful to a body that is used to a sedentary lifestyle. Any type of exercise is better than not doing any exercise at all. However, the two best exercises that have shown the best results with the least amount of effort are interval exercise and trampoline bouncing.

Interval exercise is a form of exercise of high intensity and of very short duration, which has demonstrated to raise metabolic efficiency better than other forms of exercise. It consists of performing very short periods (one to two consecutive minutes) of intense exercise (until muscular exhaustion is achieved), followed by intercalated periods of somewhat longer rest (two to three minutes).

What has been discovered is that by bringing the muscles to the point of exhaustion, the so-called growth hormone is produced, which is a musculature strengthening and regenerating hormone, which also burns fat and has a certain anti-aging effect. The growth hormone is known as "HGH" for Human Growth

Hormone, and sometimes you will see advertisements offering supplements, which claim to help increase this hormone, although there are no scientific studies to confirm this claim. The growth hormone has been used medically for children who have had poor body development, as it causes muscle growth and development even in the height of their bodies.

When you manage to exhaust the body's muscles by doing some intense exercise, for a short time, this hormone is produced naturally, and for the next twenty-four to thirty-six hours, your body will continue to burn fat and restore metabolic capacity.

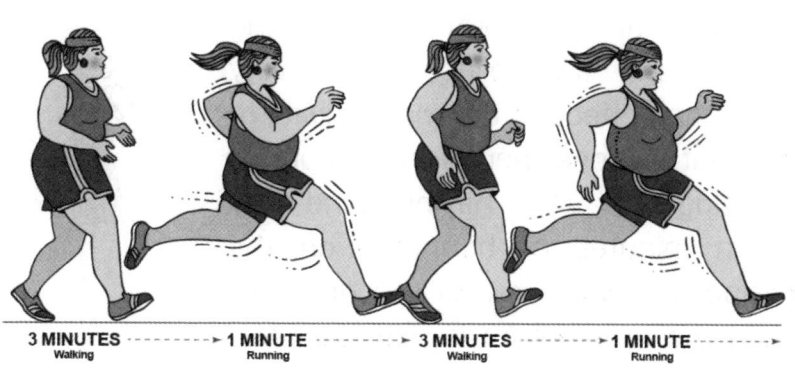

3 MINUTES Walking ----> 1 MINUTE Running ----> 3 MINUTES Walking ----> 1 MINUTE Running ---->

The concept of intense exercise for a short period of time combined with rest periods allows you to burn more fat, build more muscle and create more physical strength in just fifteen to twenty minutes of exercise than in one to two hours of long-distance walking or even long distance running.

Doing interval exercises three to four times a week, giving your body a proper routine of one day of exercise (fifteen to twenty minutes) and another day of rest without exercise, for sure will help you slim down and continue in the process of restoring your metabolism.

In my book *The Power of Your Metabolism*, I recommended the low-impact exercises that can be done on a trampoline bouncer. This type of exercise has been shown to greatly improve metabolism and has the additional benefit that it is a low impact exercise, which does not risk the person suffering damage to their knees or back, as might happen when a person chooses to jog, run, or lift weights as a form of physical exercise.

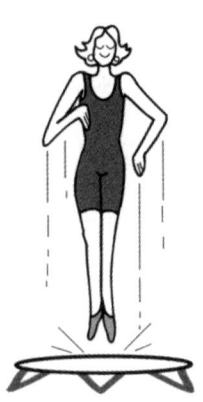

Doing fifteen minutes of bouncing on a home trampoline has a very stimulating effect on the metabolism, to the point that one spends an hour or two sweating right after having done only fifteen minutes of bouncing on the trampoline. Body sweat occurs only when the metabolism is activated and the body is heated, thus, sweating is a clear indication of a restored or activated metabolism.

The trick with the bouncing trampoline is to avoid buying the ultra-cheap models sold by Wal-Mart and other discount stores, which are very low-quality equipment models, which can even cause someone to suffer an accident while bouncing, because of the unstable structure to support the weight of the person.

Now, in sports stores, we sometimes find trampoline units that, although they have a higher cost, are well manufactured units, which use good quality tubing and springs, so they allow you to do the bouncing exercises safely and without the trampoline feeling unstable when bouncing on it. Good quality trampoline models feel heavy, have a stabilizing bar for hand support and come with a storage case.

There is an American company that sells trampolines on the internet that provides a good quality trampoline (I have one that I have been using to work out for years) that, besides being of good quality, can be folded for storage and comes with a music video with workout routines for beginners, intermediate level, and advanced rebounding routines. This company is called "Urban Rebounder" (www.urbanrebounding.com).

I have never seen an exercise that helps people slim down faster than the small trampoline bouncer. I spent many years researching the types of exercises that could help overweight or obese people, taking into consideration that these people do not possess large amounts of energy or strength.

I observed that some exercises are not appropriate for overweight people, because they are exercises that can cause impact to the knees or back, such as jogging or lifting weights. Other exercises have the main disadvantage that they are boring, such as walking on a treadmill or lifting weights. Some require spaces or very specialized equipment, such as riding a bicycle or swimming in a pool.

The small trampoline bouncer is a low-impact exercise that anyone overweight or obese can do. It doesn't require a lot of strength because the trampoline itself provides the rebound resistance. According to studies I have seen, this trampoline bouncer has the main benefit that it exercises the ENTIRE body, since the action of bouncing, and going against and then in favor of the gravity of the planet, stimulates and exercises all the cells of the body, without exception.

With this type of exercise, ALL the cells are exercised. The cells of the body, with their joint action, are the ones that generate the metabolism or energy of the body. When all of them are exercised they stimulate to raise the metabolism.

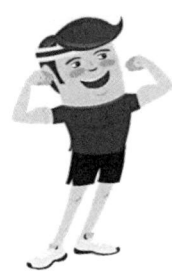

Starting to exercise on the correct gradient will guarantee you success. Just wait until you feel the energy you need to do it. Not exercising has been shown to degenerate the body's health. I do not know what you prefer, I prefer to "die with my boots on", being able to move my body and in health. Life with symptoms, body aches, pains, ailments, and dependence on a variety of medications is not very pleasant. You can decide to live life in health. Physical exercise will help you do that.

Pathway to an Ultra-Powerful Metabolism

👀 **Being in movement and doing physical exercise will ensure that we have better health and that our metabolism is fully restored.**
- You should start exercising in the correct sequence, after starting to apply the hydration, the nutrition according to your type of nervous system in the proportion of the 3x1 Diet and when you feel energetic. By applying the recommendations of this book, you will feel energy, desire to move and do exercises.
- It is important to start exercising in gradients so as not to hurt our body.
- Choose the exercise you like the most, any movement is better than nothing when it comes to restoring your metabolism.

👀 **Answer the following questions**
1. What exercise or exercises have you decided to start doing after you feel the energy to do them?

Intermittent Fasting To Help A Stuck Metabolism

When you apply the recommendations in this book, which are proven truths about how to create an Ultra-Powerful Metabolism for your body, you will undoubtedly obtain favorable results.

But you should also know that there exists a hormonal type of obstacle that affects some people's metabolism, whereby for several weeks they start slimming down well and then suddenly, for no apparent reason, they stop slimming down. The person feels as if their progress has hit a wall. In other words, their progress is stuck. This obstacle is called **INSULIN RESISTANCE.**

Consuming an excess of Type F Foods (fattening foods) creates an excess of blood glucose. Whenever there is excess GLUCOSE (blood sugar) in your body combined with excess of INSULIN the result will always be that your body will create excess FAT. This is so because the basic formula for creating fat is like this:

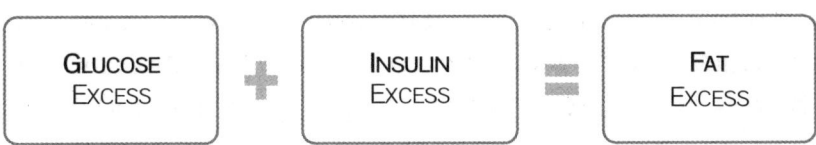

Insulin is the hormone that lowers blood glucose and does so by allowing the body's cells to use that glucose as fuel, rather than storing it as fat. When cells already have a sufficient supply of glucose, insulin is used to store the excess glucose as fat. That is why we say that insulin makes you fat.

But you should also know that if there is an excess of insulin circulating in your body, the accumulated fat will not have any way to leave the body. We could say that an excess of insulin closes the exit door to fat. The reason why the great majority of people with diabetes put on weight is precisely because they have an EXCESS OF INSULIN circulating in their body that prevents them from slimming down. If there is an excess of insulin, your body can only accumulate fat, never eliminate it.

Many of the people who are trying to slim down have already made the effort and reduced their consumption of Type F (fattening) foods, so from the beginning they noticed that their clothing size was getting smaller. But some of them notice that their body reaches a point where it simply refuses to give up the accumulated fat.

All these people started to slim down following the 3x1 Diet, good hydration, candida yeast cleansing and other recommendations in this book, but those who suddenly got stuck and stopped slimming down are unaware that they suffer from INSULIN RESISTANCE. When there is INSULIN RESISTANCE, people get stuck and when they stop slimming down, they get discouraged. Some even abandon their efforts simply because they do not know what else to do to unleash their progress.

INSULIN RESISTANCE is the result of overly consuming Type F Foods for too long, which by greatly increasing blood glucose, also forced your body to produce an EXCESS OF INSULIN. When the body's cells experience an excess of insulin, which is continuous for months or years, INSULIN RESISTANCE develops. Since an excess of insulin does not allow the body to reduce its fat reserves, you will find it exceedingly difficult or impossible to slim down.

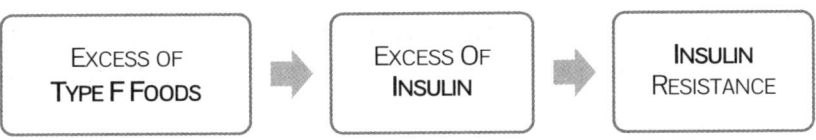

Anyone who owns a mobile phone can understand how exactly INSULIN RESISTANCE was created in the cells of your body. Let me explain using a comparison I can make between the cells in your body and your mobile phone.

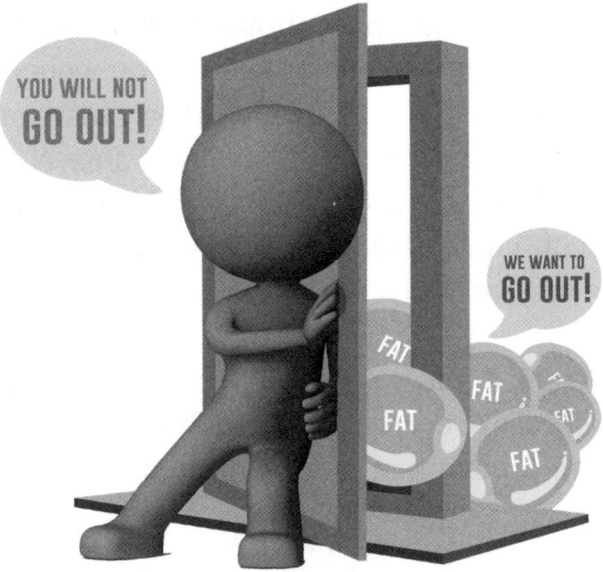

You should first know that INSULIN is a hormone, and that hormones in some ways are very much like a CALL TO YOUR CELLPHONE. Hormones, like the calls you receive, are MESSAGES that tell your cells to perform an action.

The message from the insulin hormone to the cells is one that is equivalent to "I command you to let the glucose inside you". That is, insulin commands each cell to take in the glucose that is in the blood and use it as fuel for metabolism. It is a command like the one a mother gives to their young children to get them to sit down to eat and not to get up from their chairs until they have finished eating.

Having an excess of insulin would be like having an excess of calls to your cellphone. If, for example, you receive twenty to forty calls a day on your cellphone, it could be said that you receive an abundant traffic of daily calls. But what would you do if every salesperson in your country, by mistake, had obtained your mobile phone number as a potential customer and you were receiving an avalanche of three to five hundred calls every day? What would you do to avoid having to answer so many calls from so many salespeople harassing you? Would you turn off your cellular phone? Would you apply for a different cellular phone number?

Certainly, if you were forced to receive such a high volume of calls every day, your cellphone would be totally useless as a means of communication, and you would come to hate your cellphone and the excessive calls it receives.

Well, no one can answer and comfortably handle three to five hundred calls a day. The same thing happens to the cells in your body. Every cell in your body has so-called insulin receptors on the outside, which are like tiny little antennas that receive the signal or message from the hormone insulin. These insulin receptors do the same as your cellular, they receive the messages or calls from the insulin that orders it to receive more glucose.

When there is an EXCESS OF INSULIN that constantly commands the cells to allow glucose in, to protect themselves from an excess of insulin, the cells turn off their insulin receptors. In other words, the cells ignore the signal or message from the insulin hormone just as you would if you had five hundred salesmen trying to talk to you every day.

The continuous EXCESS OF INSULIN disables the insulin receptors thus making the cells ignore insulin.

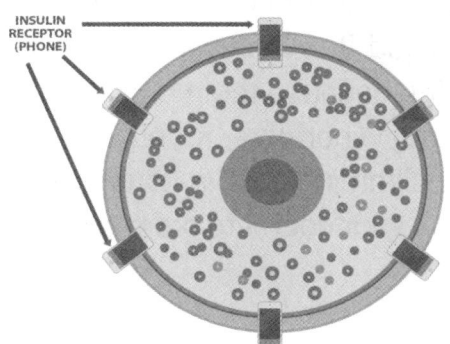

cell with functioning receptors

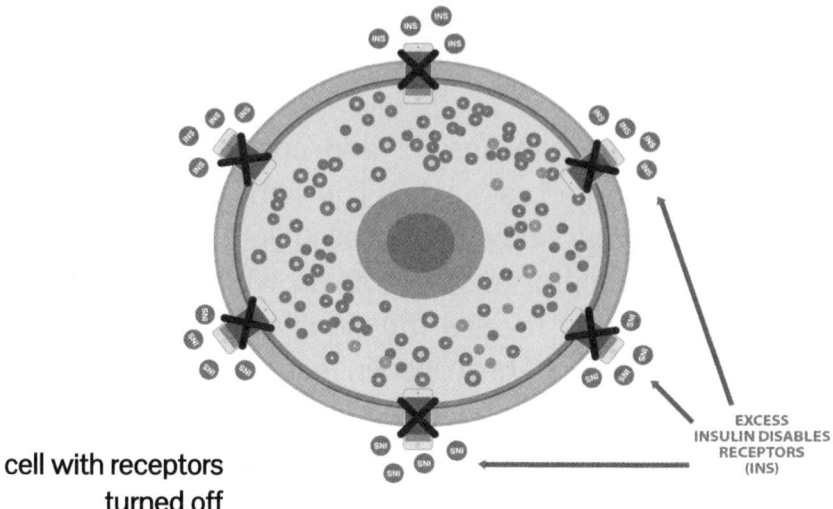

cell with receptors turned off

EXCESS INSULIN DISABLES RECEPTORS (INS)

Over-indulging in Type F Foods for many years creates a continuous excess of glucose which in turn forces the body to produce an excess of insulin. That excess of insulin inevitably develops into INSULIN RESISTANCE.

Insulin resistance is something that can be measured with a very inexpensive laboratory test that measures what is called INSULIN AT FASTING. Insulin is vital to life because without insulin the body would not be able to use glucose and the cells would die. But if there is too much insulin in the blood it will prevent the body from being able to reduce fat, because too much insulin stops the fat from coming out. Therefore, if you suspect that you have stopped slimming down due to insulin resistance, you can ask your doctor to order an INSULIN AT FASTING lab test.

Fasting Insulin Levels	
In an athlete or person in very good health	3 to 6 mIU/L (is the same as 21 to 42 pmol/L)
General population average with obesity tendency	10 to 14 mIU/L (is the same as 70 to 97 pmol/L)
mIU/L = milli-international units per liter • pmol/L = picomole per liter	

Any level of insulin at fasting that is greater than 8 mIU/L (56 pmol/L) will make it difficult for you to slim down simply because insulin will not allow fat to escape.

Insulin Resistance causes:
- high cholesterol levels
- continuous fatigue
- difficulty concentrating
- excessive hunger
- stubborn abdominal fat
- high blood pressure, as it causes the body to retain sodium, which raises blood pressure

There is a way of eating that has become trendy over the last few years, and it is called INTERMITTENT FASTING. Intermittent fasting is not a diet, it is a way of structuring the hours of the day when you give your body food and the hours of the day when you do not give your body food.

Fasting is a period of the day when you do not ingest any solid food. Drinking water, coffee, or green or vegetable juices, which are naturally low carbohydrate liquids, does not break your fast. In my research on metabolism, I found that intermittent fasting can be an excellent tool for defeating insulin resistance.

Because an excess of insulin is what caused the condition of insulin resistance, intermittent fasting works to reactivate the insulin receptors. Since biblical times different cultures have used fasting to debug[91] the body. When a person is sick, the body naturally becomes less hungry and begins to create an internal cleansing of the body that is in effect a product of involuntary fasting.

For the purposes of understanding intermittent fasting, it is necessary to think in terms of two periods of the day:

1. Period of Nourishing the Body
2. Period of Cleansing and Repairing the Body - Fasting

The hours in which our body sleeps are part of our fasting hours. So, we can say that we all fast daily while we sleep.

The key to breaking INSULIN RESISTANCE is to gradually increase the time of fasting while also gradually reducing the time of eating.

I have known hundreds of people who failed in their attempt to do intermittent fasting simply because they

---

[91] debug: to cleanse or purify.

did not prepare their body for the effort. Anyone can do intermittent fasting, but to do it you need to prepare your body.

There are events that require quite a bit of practice before they can be executed. If an athlete is preparing for a big race of hundreds of kilometers, he will have, by force and by logic, to first condition his body with practice and daily physical exercise before launching into a race that can easily exhaust him if he is not physically prepared.

To begin intermittent fasting and really succeed in breaking insulin resistance, you need to do the following:

1. Prepare your body for fasting with abundant doses of potassium and magnesium which are the two essential minerals that allow your body to store enough glucose in the liver, for the liver to serve as a reserve tank. Potassium should be used on a body weight basis. The formula we use is two capsules of potassium (each has 99 milligrams of potassium) per 11kg (25lb) of body weight. If for example a person weighs 77kg (170lb) we would know that he/she should take fourteen capsules of potassium per day:

    in kilos: 77kg divided by 11 = 7 x 2 = potassium capsules
    in pounds: 170lb divided by 25 = 7 x 2 = potassium capsules

    If the person weighs 110kg (243lb) then that would be twenty capsules of potassium per day. There is no danger from potassium for people who do not suffer from kidney disease. Get properly informed about the benefits and dosages of potassium on MetabolismoTV and clear your doubts. Watch Episode #545: Fear of Potassium.

2. You should know that without magnesium potassium cannot function. Magnesium and potassium are an inseparable duo. Magnesium should be used according to your intestinal tolerance. The dosage is increased gradually until diarrhea occurs (from the excess of magnesium) and at that point the dosage is reduced to its previous point. There are eight kinds of magnesium. The one that works best is magnesium citrate. Do not waste your time buying magnesium oxide which happens to be the least absorbed form of magnesium. Information on how to detect your correct amount of magnesium is available on MetabolismoTV. Watch Episode #1196: How Much Magnesium Should I Take.

3. Do everything possible to clear the candida albicans yeast infection before you start doing your intermittent fasting. There are many people who stop slimming down and get stuck only because their bodies are severely infected with candida yeast . A lifetime of consuming an excess of Type F Foods, which are the foods that promote candida reproduction, creates an invasive candida colony inside your body whose toxins create a slow metabolism.

When the body is heavily infected with candida yeast, and you try to do intermittent fasting, you can have a very bad time. By fasting for twelve or more hours the glucose levels are reduced, and the yeast begins to die off inside your body due to lack of glucose. At that point the excess dead and decaying yeast creates an extremely toxic environment in your blood, and you may experience the unpleasant symptoms of DETOXIFICATION (headache, diarrhea, dizziness, itchy skin, etc.).

Experiencing these candida yeast detoxification symptoms may make you think that it is the intermittent fasting that is producing these unpleasant symptoms, but the truth is different. It is not the fasting that is giving you the symptoms, it is the yeast infection and the death of the colony caused by the reduction in glucose levels. That is why within the NaturalSlim System we always have our members first clean out the candida yeast infection before attempting the intermittent fasting to overcome insulin resistance. It is not logical to try to overcome insulin resistance if you have not first removed the candida yeast infection from the body which is a major cause of slow metabolism. Watch Episode #721: How to Cure Candida Yeast Effectively.

4. Gradually increase the hours of fasting. Any period of twelve hours or more without ingesting solid

food is already a fasting period. The idea is to gradually increase the daily fasting hours (periods without food) while reducing the hours of food intake. We want to give the body a chance to gradually adapt to the reduced feeding period while increasing the fasting period. One of the most common mistakes is not giving the body enough time to adapt and this can cause you to fail in your attempt to use intermittent fasting as a method of breaking insulin resistance.

Gradual Step #	Hours fasting without solid food	Hours for food intake	Hours of the day
1	12	12	24
2	14	10	24
3	16	8	24

If you reduce the hours of feeding the body gradually you will notice that your body will adapt easily, and interestingly, you will not feel hungry during the fast. If, on the contrary, you jump in without giving the body a good preparation process, you will easily end up like most people who start intermittent fasting. They last a couple of weeks and fall apart, simply because their bodies were not prepared for intermittent fasting. Doing intermittent fasting successfully is like running a marathon; you need to prepare properly to achieve success.

It has been discovered that when you go twelve hours or more without eating your body automatically begins to cleanse and repair itself internally. When the body senses that insulin levels have been reduced, one of the internal repairs it makes in the cells is to reactivate the insulin receptors.

If there is an excess of insulin the body turns off the insulin receptors to protect itself from the excess; but if on the other hand, there is a shortage of insulin (caused by the fasting period), the body responds by doing what is necessary to activate its insulin receptors and use its main food which is glucose. This activation of the insulin receptors is a way for your body to take advantage of the little insulin that is available at the time.

5. Maintaining good hydration (always based on your body weight) during intermittent fasting and use the 3x1 Diet to portion your meals during the eating period. If you do this, plus the four recommendations above, your success will be guaranteed, and you will succeed in helping to unstock your body by breaking insulin resistance. We have proven that these five actions work for hundreds of thousands of NaturalSlim System members.

In most of the cases these five recommendations above will allow you to break INSULIN RESISTANCE to slim down and reach your goal. Certainly, with the expert help of one of NaturalSlim Certified Metabolism Consultants you could benefit from other additional aids that improve the level of results to break INSULIN RESISTANCE. There are aids to improve thyroid function, detoxify the body of candida yeast, achieve hormonal balance for men and women, plus the important aid of improving sleep quality.

Our years of experience have allowed us to learn so much about metabolism. For example, in our practice we have been able to prove, with hundreds of thousands of people, that a person will have as good results recovering their metabolism, energy or slimming as their quality of sleep. People who do not get a good night's sleep and wake up tired in the morning do not achieve their goals and become discouraged. That is why we give a lot of attention to helping NaturalSlim members to achieve a restful sleep. But if you do not have access to or do not want the help we offer at NaturalSlim, by applying these five steps you have a very good chance of effectively breaking the INSULIN RESISTANCE that keeps you from reaching your personal goal.

The obstacle of INSULIN RESISTANCE can be effectively overcome if you prepare your body properly. Most people who have tried INTERMITTENT FASTING have failed in the first few weeks simply because they did not take the necessary steps to help their body's metabolism to do so. You can succeed if you do the right things and prepare your body for the fasting period.

Pathway to an Ultra-Powerful Metabolism

∞ **Insulin Resistance does not allow you to improve your metabolism or be able to slim down.**
- Excess of insulin in the body, produced by over-consumption of refined carbohydrates, causes insulin receptors in the cells to be turned off.
- Practicing intermittent fasting helps to break insulin resistance in the body so that you can slim down.
- The five steps recommended for a successful intermittent fasting and to restore the metabolism should be followed.

∞ **Answer the following questions**
1. Describe below the steps you are already taking on your Pathway to an Ultra-Powerful Metabolism.

2. Describe how you will carry out your Intermittent Fasting if you understand that you suffer from Insulin Resistance.

THE ROAD TO RECOVERY

The data I have shared with you in this book is aimed at achieving energy and health improvements. The improvements are achieved through the application of the knowledge we have gained about how the body's metabolism works.

Ultra-Powerful Metabolism brings together the latest techniques and discoveries I have made to restore the metabolism. Remember that METABOLISM is the source of the body's ENERGY and that energy produced by the metabolism of your body's cells serves primarily to cause the MOVEMENTS we call LIFE and HEALTH. The sequence goes like this:

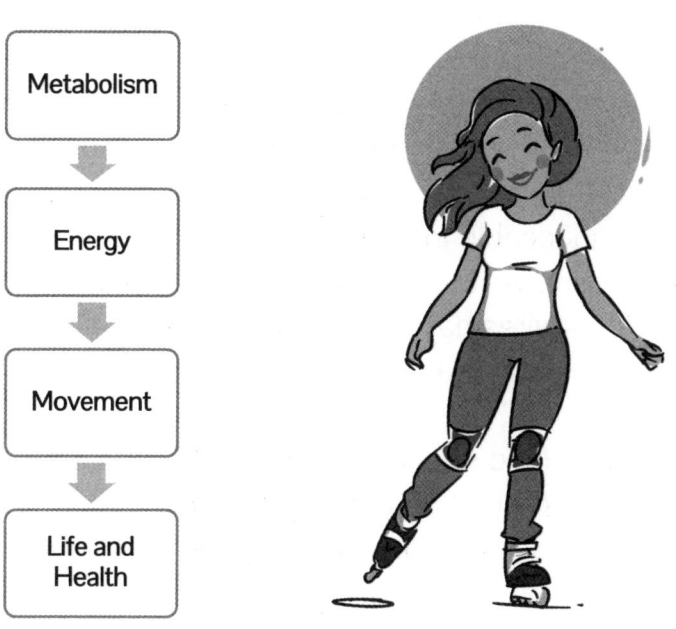

The main characteristic of LIFE is MOTION. If you want to know if something is alive or dead, you only need to observe if that something has MOTION or not. If it has MOTION, it IS ALIVE and if it does not, it is DEAD. Observe that all conditions of bad health result in a loss of movement (arthritis, cancer, obesity, etc.) while all conditions of GOOD HEALTH contain abundant MOVEMENT (exercise, dancing, gymnastics). When metabolism is restored, ENERGY is restored and that energy, when abundant, allows for a great deal of MOVEMENT which represents LIFE and HEALTH.

When you observe a very young child and notice that he or she is bursting with energy and that he or she simply never seems to get tired, you are closely observing what is a state of Ultra-Powerful Metabolism. We adults are losing energy and mobility. Children seem to have inexhaustible energy.

By applying the knowledge in this book, you put yourself on the path to recovering your body's optimal metabolic potential. If you do things correctly you will have a noticeable increase in your body's energy levels. You will have a much greater desire to exercise and enjoy life. Life requires having enough energy available for you to achieve your goals.

You should know that your body can be restored to an optimal state of abundant and vibrant energy. But it is a gradual process. It does not happen overnight.

All the cells that make up your body are alive and a cell that is defective cannot be repaired. That is, those cells in your body that were born weak because you did not eat the right nutrients, because you did not properly hydrate your body or because you had carelessly neglected your lifestyle can not be repaired. The cells that make up your body right now will be in the state of good health or poor health that each of them is currently in. The cells of your body are like a tree that if it was born crooked there is nothing you can do to straighten it out. The only way to restore the total health of the body is to make sure that the new cells that are born have available the necessary elements (vitamins, minerals, fats, proteins, carbohydrates) that they need to create NEW HEALTHY CELLS.

If you are going to build a house and the only thing you have as construction material is mud, surely your whole house will be built with mud. But if you are going to build a house and you have at your disposition good quality materials such as cement, stone, marble, and steel, you will be able to build a mansion of very high quality. The same goes for the cells of your body. If you start today to give your body good nutrition, which serves as building materials to create new cells, your body will build new cells that will be very healthy.

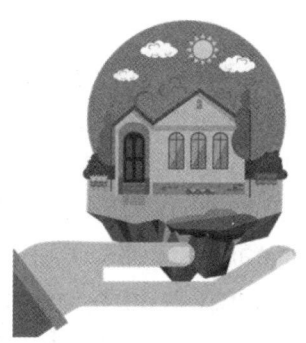

With what you provide your body today in terms of foods and <u>cell building materials, your body can not repair the cells that have already been built with the materials you previously provided your body</u>. However, your body can create new healthy cells to replace the defective cells that were born before.

What I mean by this is that the road to recovery takes a while, but it is a safe road where your body can only get better as it replaces those cells that were defective and weak with new cells that have a healthy metabolism.

Every part of the body has its own life cycle. Some cells have a short life span and are replaced quickly, and other cells have a much longer life span, so they take longer to replace.

The lifespan of each type of cell in your body is different and knowing this will allow you to calculate how long it may take to recover the maximum cellular health of each part of your body. A healthy body is composed of healthy cells. A body that is sick, weak and without energy is composed of cells that are in bad shape and you will have to wait for those cells to be replaced by new cells that have been well nourished to finally achieve a totally healthy body.

We live in a high-tech culture where we expect everything to be instantaneous, but inside the human body cells do not work like that. Each cell is born, grows and dies in its predetermined time and if the cell was born weak it will have to grow and reach its natural death while still weak. Each type of cell in the body has a specific life span and the table below will help you estimate the recovery time or what would be the extension or duration of its road to recovery.

Organ or Gland	Time	Notes
	Life Span of Cells	
eyes	2 days	Every two days we have "new eyes". That is why people who reduce their glucose levels improve their eyesight.
intestine	3 days	Every three days we will have a new intestine where defective cells are replaced by new cells.
skin	6 weeks	Every six weeks the skin is totally regenerated.
liver	8 weeks	Every eight weeks the liver is regenerated and rebuilt.
nervous system	8 months	Every eight months the cells of the nervous system and brain are replaced by new cells.
bones	15 months	Every fifteen months the bones are renewed and are completely replaced by new bone cells.

Source: Book "Healing is Voltage" by Dr. Jerry Tennat

In conclusion, if you can sustain yourself long enough on the road to recovery, by living a good lifestyle, eating the right foods for your type of nervous system, getting the necessary nutrients (vitamins and minerals) and good hydration along with an exercise regimen, and while avoiding those "toxic personalities" that sometimes create unnecessary stress, it is SURE that you will recover as much of your energy level and health as possible.

The road to recovery is more of a long-distance marathon than a short run. By following this pattern, I have seen that EVERYONE can get better if they stay on track and do not give in to the temptations of sweet addiction or refined carbohydrates. With the information in this book, *Ultra-Powerful Metabolism*, and the videos I have created for you on my MetabolismoTV YouTube channel, a path of continuous improvement awaits you if you really want to achieve it.

Pathway to an Ultra-Powerful Metabolism

👓 **Already affected cells in our body cannot be repaired. The solution is to do things the right way so that new body cells are born healthy.**
- Each type of body cell has a specific life span.
- We must remain persistent in our new lifestyle to provide enough time for the body to create new healthy cells.

👓 **Answer the following questions**
1. Calculate how long it will take you to create new healthy cells throughout your body. What actions will you take now that you know how long the road to recovery will take?

Personal Program For An Ultra-Powerful Metabolism

While you were reading the book, you answered certain questions in each chapter. Some of these questions were marked with the following symbol 🏃. The answers to these questions will complete your **Personalized Program**. You can complete your program here, rewriting the answers to the questions in the sequence below and by doing so, you would have created your Personalized Program.

STEP #1: **Establish your correct goal.**

• My goal in clothing size or waist measurement is:

• My health goal is:

STEP #2: **Hydrate your body** with the correct amount of water, according to your body weight.

• According to my body weight, I should consume _____ glasses of water daily.

STEP #3: **Identify which is your Type of Nervous System.**
• My Type of Nervous System type is:

STEP #4: **Start eating in proportion to the 3x1 Diet and according to your type of nervous system.**
• Describe how you will apply the 3x1 Diet to your breakfast, lunch, and dinner according to your type of nervous system.

STEP #5: **Calm your Nervous System.**
• Describe the actions you will take to help your nervous system and calm it down.

STEP #6: **Do the refined carbohydrates detox** so you can break the addiction and guarantee your success.
- Prepare for your Detox. Describe what foods you will be preparing for breakfast, lunch and dinner that apply to your type of nervous system during your refined carbohydrates detox.

STEP #7: **Be sure to improve your quality of sleep.**
- Describe what actions you will take to ensure that you really do get a restful night's sleep and sleep at least seven hours a day.

STEP #8: **Cleanse from the candida albicans yeast.**
- Describe what decisions you made regarding the proliferation of candida yeast in your body and what actions you will take about it.

STEP #9: **Identify if your thyroid gland is functioning well or if you are suffering from subclinical hypothyroidism.**
> • Describe the actions you will take to improve the functioning of your thyroid gland.

STEP #10: **Identify which foods may be attacking your body.**
> • Describe the actions you will take to manage the issue of Aggressor Foods.

STEP #11: **Identify if you are suffering from any hormonal imbalance.**
> • Describe what actions you will take to manage the hormonal imbalance in your body.

STEP #12: **Start exercising.**
- What exercise(s) will you start doing and how often?

STEP #13: **Start INTERMITTENT FASTING.** *This is an optional step if you understand that you are suffering from insulin resistance.
- Describe how you will carry out Intermittent Fasting if you suffer from insulin resistance.

STEP #14: **Determine how long it will take to renew all the cells in your body.**
- Describe how long it will take your entire body to recover and what actions you will take regarding recovery.

If you think you need additional assistance, please contact one of our Certified Metabolism Consultants at your nearest NaturalSlim. You can see a complete list of locations where we offer service toward the end of this book.

References and Additional Aids

NATURAL SUPPLEMENTS TO HELP YOUR METABOLISM

CANDIDA YEAST CLEANSING, CANDISEPTIC KIT

The candida albicans yeast began to take prominence as a causing factor of slow metabolism, since Dr. C. Orian Truss published his first articles on this yeast. In fact, much of the success that the NaturalSlim System has had in helping thousands of people slim down, even though many of them had already failed in their previous diets, was due to the candida yeast cleansing program. Restoration of metabolism depends on clearing this yeast from the body. As described by Dr. Truss and later by allergist Dr. William Crook in his book *The Yeast Connection*, the candida yeast creates a toxic environment within the body that reduces metabolism and causes obesity and a shocking array of other symptoms.

After their initial yeast cleanse, we always recommend that all our members do a maintenance yeast cleanse at least every six months because we have found that this helps them maintain their metabolism and body weight. Also, for diabetic patients, periodic fungal cleansing keeps them on less medications.

Cleansing of the candida yeast can produce some not very pleasant manifestations, known as the "Herxheimer syndrome", named after the physician who described the toxic state that occurs when parasitic organisms die within a body. This must be known in order to be prepared.

When the yeast die, due to the fungicidal (yeast -killing) action of the anti-candida program, they rot inside the body, and this generates toxins that can cause some temporary unpleasant manifestations, such as headache, itchy skin and others (see chapter THE CANDIDA ALBICANS YEAST).

Cleansing brings many benefits, it greatly improves the efficiency of your metabolism, and helps you slim down, plus a huge number of strange symptoms disappear. However, it is not worth trying to cleanse candida yeast if you do not first hydrate your body and start eating the 3x1 Diet. Trying to kill candida yeast while maintaining high glucose levels is a waste of time, effort, and money.

The basic strategy for reducing yeast in the body is to first weaken them by reducing their supply of glucose (their favorite food) and then kill them. It has already been discovered that the candida yeast depends on having an abundant supply of glucose for its reproduction and tissue invasion.

We discovered that when a person can reduce the amount of candida yeast in their body, their metabolism speeds up and they are able to slim down much faster and with more permanent results; that is, they do not tend to "bounce back" (lose weight and then gain it back). Therefore, an integral part of the NaturalSlim program, to help people slim down, is the candida yeast cleanse.

There is no way to eliminate 100% of the candida yeast, because this yeast is a normal inhabitant of the intestinal flora and of the vaginal flora. The goal of the yeast cleansing program is to REDUCE THE YEAST COLONY, to reduce the toxins it produces, and to restore the metabolism.

Since some people are not members of the NaturalSlim System and others who do not need our help because they do not suffer from obesity, but who wish to fight the infection of this yeast in their bodies, we created the CANDISEPTIC KIT, which is a program that contains three natural supplements to reduce the infection of the candida yeast.

This yeast cleansing program, CANDISEPTIC KIT, comes with instructions on how to use it and takes twenty-eight days to complete, because you must gradually increase the daily doses of the natural fungicide supplements that kill the yeast, as explained in the instructions. The idea of gradually increasing the doses is to lessen the unpleasant manifestations that may occur as the yeast dies inside the body.

The regular anti-candida program we use for NaturalSlim members uses more potent natural supplements (other than CANDISEPTIC), so while it achieves a more complete cleanse, it has the potential to produce unpleasant reactions that may be more serious and require assistance. For this reason, we only deliver it under the supervision of one of our Metabolism Consultants, at NaturalSlim centers, and only to members whom we monitor at weekly consultations. However, the CANDISEPTIC KIT, although of a more limited potency, can be of great help for the benefits it brings to cleanse the body of yeast, to restore metabolism. To effectively reduce the candida yeast, it is not enough to kill it, it is also necessary to replace the intestinal flora that naturally fights it and prevents the yeast from invading the body again.

The diarrhea symptoms that often occur after antibiotic treatment is caused by the death of the good bacteria that make up the body's natural intestinal flora. It is for this reason that the anti-candida program CANDISEPTIC KIT, contains a supplement of natural bacteria called probiotics that help replace the body's natural good bacteria that make up the intestinal and vaginal flora.

The candida albicans yeast is a parasite that severely infects people who have abused the consumption of refined carbohydrates, people suffering from obesity and diabetics. Reducing the fungal colony with the help of a diet that cuts down refined carbohydrates, such as the 3x1 Diet, plus reducing the fungal colony that infects the body with the help of natural supplements such as the CANDISEPTIC KIT program, is a wonderful aid in restoring metabolism.

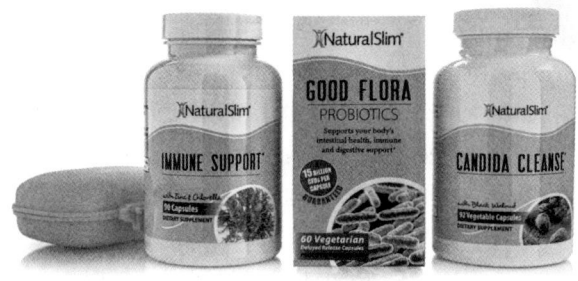

Coco-10 Plus

For more than twenty years, NaturalSlim centers have been helping thousands of people to slim down by educating them on how to improve their body's metabolism. The vast majority of those who visit us suffer from obesity. Many of them claim that they have tried everything from dieting to exercise. Many of them tell us that they had managed to slim down and soon after they put it all back on again. All of them suffer from a slow metabolism that does not allow them to slim down, and if they slim down while dieting, they put on weight again shortly after.

One of the supplements that helps us the most to restore the metabolism of thousands of people, is organic coconut oil, in our formulation called Coco-10 Plus. This formula, which combines the properties of organic coconut oil with the metabolism benefits of CoQ10 coenzyme, is a powerful oil that accelerates the process of reducing body fat.

Even after more than twenty years of using coconut oil in NaturalSlim, a great majority of physicians and nutritionists are unaware of the benefits of this wonderful substance. This happens while the official mass propaganda to reduce calories and reduce fat, only resulted in getting the population to increase their consumption of refined carbohydrates and starches, Type F Foods, which are the same foods that create the epidemics of obesity and diabetes. In the matter of trying to reduce obesity or trying to control diabetes by counting calories, it could be said that "the shot backfired".

The so-called medium-chain triglycerides in coconut oil are saturated fats that speed up metabolism, helps slim down, suppress a person's hunger and stabilize blood glucose levels. An impressive number of clinical studies provide evidence that saturated fats, especially the medium-chain triglycerides in coconut oil present no health hazards, only benefits.

It is interesting to note that consuming coconut oil lowers your triglyceride (blood fat) levels. Having a high triglyceride level in the blood is much more dangerous than having high cholesterol. Interestingly, although coconut oil is a triglyceride, it has the property that, being a medium chain oil, it is used without the help of the digestive system. It is already known that coconut oil has the property of reducing triglycerides in the blood. The regular use of coconut oil reduces abdominal obesity and insulin resistance, which is characterized by a protruding belly.

Coconut oil also has a proven antibacterial action. In fact, the lauric acid that makes up almost 50% of coconut oil works as a natural antibiotic. As you can see, coconut oil has nothing but good benefits. Whatever you have heard against coconut oil, it has been propaganda generated by some private interest, who does not want people to know that coconut oil can be a more than efficient solution to improve metabolism and health.

People who suffer from obesity or diabetes, because of their condition, have severe candida albicans yeast infections in their bodies. Because they are so infected with the candida yeast, it is VERY IMPORTANT that the dosage of COCO-10 PLUS be increased very, very, gradually. Organic coconut oil has a very powerful fungicidal (yeast killing) function. Daily doses of coconut oil should be increased little by little, to give the body a chance to eliminate the toxins that are formed as the fungi die inside your body. As the fungi die, toxins form inside the body (fungal decay) and usually cause symptoms that can be very unpleasant. These are symptoms of detoxification such as headache, itchy skin, muscle pain, diarrhea, weakness due to excess toxins and others that may occur.

Years of over-consumption of refined carbohydrates, starches, sugar, or alcohol contribute to systemic (all over the body) candida yeast infections. You should try to protect your body from the toxins that form when we try to do a cleansing and detoxifying job to reduce the invading candida albicans yeast colony from the body. Coconut oil kills the candida yeast, which is why you should increase your daily dosage gradually, to avoid problems with severe detoxification symptoms. If the up dosing of tablespoons of oil is done too quickly, the symptoms may be so unpleasant that they force you to abandon the idea of trying to reduce the candida yeast infection. Here is an example of how to gradually increase the doses of COCO-10 PLUS.

First Week:
    Sunday - ½ tablespoon per day
    Monday - ½ tablespoon per day
    Tuesday - ½ tablespoon per day
    Wednesday - ½ tablespoon per day
    Thursday - ½ tablespoon per day
    Friday - ½ tablespoon per day
    Saturday - ½ tablespoon per day

Second Week:
    Sunday - 1 tablespoon per day
    Monday - 1 tablespoon per day
    Tuesday - 1 tablespoon per day
    Wednesday - 1 tablespoon per day
    Thursday - 1 tablespoon per day

Friday - 1 tablespoon per day
Saturday - 1 tablespoon per day

Third Week:
Sunday - 1 ½ tablespoon per day
Monday - 1 ½ tablespoon per day
Tuesday - 1 ½ tablespoon per day
Wednesday - 1 ½ tablespoon per day
Thursday - 1 ½ tablespoon per day
Friday - 1 ½ tablespoon per day
Saturday - 1 ½ tablespoon per day

From 1½ tablespoon a day, the dose would be increased to 2 tablespoons a day, and so on, based on ½ tablespoon increase, for each week. You can continue to increase the dose up to a maximum of four tablespoons a day if your body allows it. If your body begins to have more or less constant diarrhea (this happens when too many yeasts die at once), you have gone over the correct dosage for your body and you should reduce it. Most people do very well with two tablespoons a day. Note that we are talking about tablespoons, not teaspoons.

Coco-10 Plus helps to reduce the candida albicans yeast in the body, and that gets your metabolism up, which will help you slim down. However, it is important that you increase the dosage of Coco-10 Plus gradually, to give your body a chance to eliminate the toxins produced by killing the yeast in your body. Coco-10 Plus can be taken straight by mouth in spoonful because it does not really have a taste. But typically, you increase the dose each week by ½ tablespoon, which can be added to a protein shake that you prepare in the morning.

Constipend For Constipation

For anyone interested in improving their metabolism to slim down, it is very important that their body can have a normal transit time between the time they eat food and the time they eliminate waste. At NaturalSlim we have found that anyone who suffers from constipation will not be able to achieve their goal until they are able to regulate their bowel movements. This makes a lot of sense when we realize that the word metabolism originates from the Greek word *meta* which means MOVEMENT. Metabolism has everything to do with the movements of the body. A congested bowel, not moving at the right speed, is a clear indication of slow metabolism.

Going to the bathroom, at least once a day, is the reasonable minimum, and the ideal would be to have a natural elimination, two to three times a day. When this does not happen, the walls of the intestine gradually fill with a sticky and resinous layer that hinders the absorption of nutrients. Especially if the person is not accustomed to consuming enough water daily, the feces become compacted against the walls of the intestine and congestion occurs, which not only hinders absorption, but creates an extremely toxic state in the body, which in turn contributes to a slow metabolism.

When the body is excessively toxic due to the accumulation of feces on the walls of the intestine, the metabolism is reduced, and the person will not be able to slim down. In these cases, problems with hemorrhoids, allergies or skin problems often start to appear, simply because the body is excessively toxic, due to intestinal congestion.

The main cause of cellulite or orange-peel skin on the buttocks or hips, which distresses women so much and creates a million-dollar market for creams, liposuction, and a multitude of other remedies, is constipation and the accumulation of waste and feces that impact the walls of the intestine. In short, the intestine becomes a clogged pipe that accumulates toxins and creates an environment conducive to bacteria, fungi, and parasites.

I do not recommend the repeated and regular use of laxatives because they work by irritating the delicate bowel tissue, as do supplements based on *cascara sagrada*. (also known by the names California buckthorn, bearberry, yellow bark, and sacred bark). CONSTIPEND decongests, cleanses, and helps regenerate the intestinal tissues without causing irritation. When used along with MAGICMAG magnesium powder, even the most difficult cases of constipation are resolved, since most of the population is deficient in magnesium, which is one of the main causes of constipation.

To have good metabolism, it is necessary to avoid the accumulation of toxins in the intestine, achieving an adequate intestinal movement, and for that purpose CONSTIPEND can be of great help.

Natural Progesterone Femme Balance

To help women with hormonal balance we use the natural progesterone cream FEMME BALANCE. To function properly, the human metabolism needs to maintain a balance in both the hormonal system and the nervous system of the body.

The body of a woman is designed to ensure the reproduction of the race, so the hormonal system of a woman is much more complex than that of a man. The fat content of a woman's body must always be higher than a man's, simply because fat is the most efficient way to store energy that can be used later by the body to produce breast milk. Breast milk is high in its caloric fat content, so a woman's body is designed to always have more fat available than a man's body. It is completely normal for a woman's body weight to be composed of 30% fat while that of men is around 20%. So, the higher proportion of fat in a woman's body is a matter of divine design. To top it off, it is estimated that men's bodies contain 25% more muscle (which burns fat) than women's bodies. The composition chart, which compares a man's body to a woman's as well, reflects that women's bodies naturally contain up to 80% more fat than men's bodies.

For the above reasons, women always need more help slimming down than men because their bodies are naturally designed to store fat. For example, among the members of the NaturalSlim System, who receive our weekly slim down consulting, on average 85% are women and only 15% are men. Women need much more assistance in restoring metabolism than men largely because of the hormonal difference that causes their bodies to produce much more of the female estrogen hormone (fattening hormone) than the male testosterone hormone (slim down and muscle building hormone).

It is easy to see that the estrogen hormone is fattening. Women who at one time or another used birth control pills or hormone replacement medications such as Premarin and Prempro, among others, could not avoid gaining weight. Both birth control pills and hormone replacement medications that have been used for women in menopause are made from the estrogen hormone. Estrogen accumulates fat. In addition to its fat-accumulating effect, it is already known that estrogen can be a cause and promoting agent (accelerating the growth) of breast cancer. For that reason, when a woman is found to have breast cancer, doctors always recommend that all sources of estrogen be eliminated.

To restore metabolism, it is necessary to reduce obesity, but to reduce obesity it is also necessary to reduce or counteract the predominance of estrogen. The estrogen hormone is closely linked to obesity in women. Natural progesterone has the effect of counteracting excess estrogen, which is why it helps women slim down. This has been our experience in more than twenty years of using the natural progesterone supplement FEMME BALANCE in NaturalSlim centers.

Natural progesterone has other benefits for women. For example, natural progesterone has the effect of maintaining the skin's natural moisture and makes a woman's skin acquire a youthful luster. In the field of aesthetics, where facial or body treatments are performed, progesterone is considered an anti-aging hormone.

An additional effect of progesterone is that it raises the libido (desire for sexual activity) in women. The husbands of many of the women participating in the NaturalSlim slimming down system who already supplement with the natural progesterone cream FEMME BALANCE comment that they have noticed the difference.

One subject to clarify, for the sake of truth, is the confusion that exists in the medical field between PROGESTERONE and PROGESTINS. Natural progesterone has only positive effects; it even helps prevent breast cancer by counteracting excess estrogen. **Progestins manufactured by the pharmaceutical industry are not the same as natural progesterone.** Progestins are a form of SYNTHETIC [92] PROGESTERONE that simply cannot be the same as natural progesterone because it could not be patented.

Pharmaceutical companies feel obliged to protect their large economic investments in drug development, so they cannot use any natural product as part of their formulations. A natural product CANNOT BE PATENTED. If it cannot be patented, it cannot be commercially protected from possible copying by competitors. Therefore, the solution of the pharmaceutical companies has been to create PROGESTINS which are bad synthetic copies of natural progesterone.

None of the pharmaceuticals use NATURAL PROGESTERONE, they only use PROGESTINS, which are chemical and synthetic imitations of natural progesterone. Because they are chemicals that are not natural to the body, progestins cause side effects and do not have the cancer protective effect or any of the other benefits that natural progesterone has. Some

---

[92] synthetic: a synthetic medication is one composed of substances manufactured by the pharmaceutical industry that are not natural to the body.

physicians, who have not explored the subject, commonly and mistakenly, call pharmaceutical medications made with PROGESTIN progesterone. Medications with PROGESTIN have a very bad history of causing breast cancer, which is why several clinical studies had to be cancelled when it was discovered that women were getting too many cases of breast cancer when using PROGESTIN. Natural progesterone has nothing to do with the progestins that were found to cause cancer in the studies that had to be cancelled.

So, use FEMME BALANCE natural progesterone because it works. I do not like the theory; I like POSITIVE RESULTS. I share with you all that I have learned about these subjects and invite you to explore for yourself the validity of what I explain here. Metabolism can be restored; to do so requires KNOWLEDGE that has not necessarily been available before.

DIGESTIVE ENZYMES HELPZYMES

The body's digestive system transforms the food we eat (proteins, carbohydrates, fats, vitamins, minerals) into nutrients in simpler forms, which our metabolism can convert into energy. Without this transformation by digestion, neither the assimilation nor the utilization of nutrients would be possible to allow the continuous creation of energy that maintains health.

Your body's metabolism will create the body's energy efficiently, only if digestion does not fail to transform the food you ate. For example, a piece of chicken breast can be a good source of protein. However, that protein called "chicken breast" has to first be digested and then transformed from protein to amino acid before it can be assimilated by the cells, so that the body can then use it to create energy. If digestion fails, metabolism will fail.

The foods you choose and then consume in your diet are your body's combustible, just as gasoline is the combustible for your car's engine. If the gasoline does not efficiently reach your car's engine, where combustion will occur with the help of oxygen, your car will run out of energy to move the wheels. Likewise, if the food you eat is not digested and absorbed well, the energy produced by your metabolism will be reduced and so will your overall health. We have proven that among obese and diabetic people digestive problems (acidity, reflux, gas, tiredness, or sleepiness after eating, indigestion, etc.) are very common.

To restore your metabolism, it is necessary to make sure that the food is digested and assimilated correctly, because otherwise, it would be like having problems with the car engine, due to defects in the engine carburetor, which is the equipment that does the vital work of distributing gasoline to the engine.

It can be a waste of time and money if you try to choose good quality foods (organic, whole foods, fresh foods, etc.) if your body has digestive problems, which cause it to not take advantage of them. To have a good metabolism you also need to have good digestion!

There is a common saying that "you are what you eat" but although this sounds logical, it is not actually true. Rather than "you are what you eat" the reality is that "you are what you digest". If you do not digest a food well, the body will not be able to use it. You may choose the foods in your diet very well, however, the nutrients will not be assimilated by the cells of your body if digestion is impaired.

Every time you eat something, and your body tells you that there are digestive problems with gas, burping, flatulence, acidity, your body is telling you: I could not digest it! I am sorry to tell you this, but everything that is not digested, rots inside the body.

Many of the people seeking our help to restore their metabolism suffer from these digestive problems, which is why we had to develop a specialized digestive enzyme supplement, called HELPZYMES; to help them with their digestion and thus improve the efficiency of their body's metabolism.

The problem of digestion is made worse when the person suffers from hypothyroidism (lazy thyroid), since this thyroid condition, in addition to a slow metabolism and obesity, can cause many people to be unable to digest their food well, due to a lack of a good production of hydrochloric acid (HCL[93]) produced in the stomach. It is known that there is a close relationship between hypothyroidism and deficient production of hydrochloric acid in the stomach. Hydrochloric acid is a very strong acid that the stomach produces so that you can digest even the most difficult to digest proteins.

Many people who take antacid medications suffer from acidity because their body does not produce enough hydrochloric acid, so what they eat decomposes in their stomach or intestine. Everything that decomposes, rots, and as it rots, it becomes acidic. When a food breaks down,

---

[93] HCL (hydrochloric acid): acid produced by the stomach as part of its gastric juices to digest food.

because it cannot be digested due to lack of hydrochloric acid, it produces stomach acidity, which can sometimes be mistaken for "excess acid", when in fact it is exactly the opposite: lack of sufficient hydrochloric acid to digest proteins.

Hypochlorhydria[94] is a condition estimated by some to affect more than fifty percent of people over the age of sixty, in which gastric acid production in the stomach is deficient or low.

It is interesting that many people who come to NaturalSlim with obesity and acidity problems arrive taking antacid medications such as Prevacid, Zegerid, Prilosec, Zantac, Protonix and many others. However, by spending just a couple of weeks, accompanying their meals with HELPZYMES digestive enzymes, and while hydrating their body daily with plenty of water, almost 100% of them no longer need to continue using their antacid medications.

Hypochlorhydria (acid deficiency in gastric juices) has been ignored, mainly because it is very difficult to diagnose. Conveniently, by ignoring this digestive problem, a giant market has been created for pharmaceutical companies to sell over the counter and prescription antacid medications. The public is simply unaware of this subject, so they live in dependence on antacids, while suffering from very bad digestion.

The solution to the problem of acidity is affordable and permanent, because even HELPZYMES enzymes, in many

---

[94] hypochlorhydria: a condition in which the stomach has a deficient production of hydrochloric acid (HCL), which causes indigestion that develops into stomach acidity. The manifestations are almost identical to those of gastroesophageal reflux for which several other medications are also promoted.

cases do not have to be used permanently, once the normal digestion process is restored, with the help of the 3x1 Diet, plus good hydration. The body has a great capacity for recovery when it is well treated.

The gastric juices of the stomach have many other functions in addition to those of digestion. One of them is to serve as a barrier to infectious or parasitic organisms that may be hidden in food. Having a good production of gastric juices prevents infectious diseases. Even infections with the famous bacteria "helicobacter pylori" [95], which is blamed for the stomach ulcers of millions of people, have to do with the deficient production of hydrochloric acid, which is an important part of gastric juices.

HELPZYMES digestive enzymes include a moderate dose of hydrochloric acid to assist the person in digesting their food. Nevertheless, the most important components of the HELPZYMES supplement are the enzymes that digest proteins, fats, and carbohydrates. One of the most important digestive enzymes is called pancrelipase, which is an enzyme produced by the pancreas (where insulin is also produced). Pancrelipase, which contains a combination of three enzymes: amylase to digest carbohydrates, trypsin to digest proteins and lipase to digest fats. HELPZYMES digestive enzymes are fortified with pancrelipase because we have seen it dramatically improve digestion in those suffering from obesity or diabetes.

When formulating HELPZYMES enzymes, I realized that the digestive enzyme supplement industry was full of unethical

---

[95] helicobacter pylori bacteria: bacteria that lives exclusively in the human stomach. It is a spiral bacterium (its shape resembles the blades of a helicopter) which is why it acquired its name "helicobacter". Indeed, its spiral shape allows it to penetrate and screw itself into the stomach wall, which is why it is accused of being the cause of stomach ulcers.

offerings, in the sense that some manufacturers claimed to offer digestive enzymes without being able to prove the ACTIVITY of those enzymes. They tried to sell digestive enzymes "by weight", which is completely illogical, since it is not the weight or amount of an enzyme that achieves good digestion, but its proven activity to digest proteins, carbohydrates, or fats.

After an intense search, I found more reliable manufacturers who could provide us with laboratory analysis certifying the level of digestive activity their enzymes had. Even in the field of natural products there is a money motive, which often causes product offerings that promise help that they cannot deliver.

People who do not digest their food well come to develop a bad odor in the sweat of their bodies, which is caused by protein and other indigestible foods inside their body. Once digestion is fixed, acidity disappears, along with the other manifestations of digestive problems, such as gases, belching, flatulence, excessive sleepiness after eating, and bad body odor. In addition, metabolism is greatly improved, which is noted in reduced body fat, improved energy level and improved diabetes control.

Digestion is a VITAL process that determines the difference between good or bad health. To restore metabolism and slim down, you must have good digestion.

Potassium Kadsorb

The best way to supplement with potassium is to drink fresh vegetable juices and leafy green juices (spinach, lettuce, etc.), the kind that are prepared with a juice extractor because that way the natural potassium content of the vegetables is made available to the body, along with the rest of the nutrients. Nothing works better than supplementation with fresh vegetable juices.

If there is no kidney (renal) condition, generally there will be no reasonable medical objection against supplementing the diet with a small or moderate dose of potassium capsules. Potassium capsules or tablets are manufactured in doses of 99 milligrams each in most countries. An 8-ounce (237 milliliter) carrot juice contains about 600 milligrams of potassium (equivalent to six capsules) and a medium-sized plantain (banana) contains about 400 milligrams of potassium (equal to four capsules). To think that consuming four or six capsules of potassium a day can harm someone whose kidney function is not impaired is equivalent to thinking that consuming a carrot juice or a banana could harm us. There is no danger in supplementing with potassium capsules or tablets if the renal (kidney) function is in good condition.

The total recommended daily intake of potassium per person is 4,700 milligrams per day, according to the National Institute of Medicine. However, the problem is that the general population consumes too much sodium (estimated to be over 4,000 milligrams per day) and too little potassium (estimated to be about 2,300 milligrams), instead of the recommended 4,700 milligrams. People simply do not consume enough VEGETABLES and GREEN SALAD to meet their bodies' potassium needs. That is the real problem!

Potassium is an essential mineral that maintains the balance of water in the body besides being used by the body to neutralize acids, both in the blood and inside the cells. It is also essential for muscle building and for the transmission of electrical signals in our nervous system. Symptoms of potassium deficiency, called hypokalemia (too low potassium), can be as follows:

- ☐ anxiety, nervousness
- ☐ leg cramps
- ☐ mental confusion
- ☐ muscular weakness
- ☐ depression
- ☐ sugar or sweet cravings
- ☐ memory impairment
- ☐ muscle spasms
- ☐ fatigue
- ☐ sodium intolerance
- ☐ irritability
- ☐ very dry skin
- ☐ slow reflexes
- ☐ liquid retention
- ☐ restless legs syndrome

One of the easiest symptoms to detect potassium deficiency is cramps. These leg cramps, which can be so painful and are usually worse at night, can be solved by supplementing with potassium capsules, such as KADSORB.

The body cannot use glucose without the help of potassium. In fact, when potassium is depleted, one of the effects caused is an unusual rise in blood glucose. Potassium deficiencies reduce glucose utilization, thus increasing blood glucose levels. Therefore, diuretic medications used to lower hypertension, which also have the effect of reducing potassium in the body, increase glucose in diabetics and non-diabetics. If there is a deficiency of potassium or magnesium, which allows the cells to use potassium, it is not possible to restore metabolism.

The intake of potassium in the diet should be much higher than that of sodium, as recommended by the National Institute of Medicine itself. However, the current ratio of potassium to sodium consumption is the opposite of what it should be, which is why there is an epidemic of people suffering from high blood pressure. The references on the relationship between excessive sodium consumption and hypertension are more than clear. On the other hand, the scientific references on the ability of potassium supplementation to reduce blood pressure in patients who do not have renal problems also leave no doubt.

The right thing to do, in addition to asking patients with hypertension to reduce their sodium intake, would be to help patients reduce their blood pressure by supplementing their diet with potassium to counteract the excess sodium in their diets. Hopefully, we could get all people with hypertension to consume much more vegetables and green salad in their diets. Fruits have a good potassium content, but for the most part, except for strawberries and apples, they are too high in fructose, and that brings its own problems.

Same as with the different types of magnesium, potassium also comes in different forms (citrate, gluconate, chloride, etc.), and some forms of potassium are more absorbable than others. In the case of NaturalSlim, we chose potassium citrate for our KADSORB supplement. It turned out that potassium citrate proved to be the most absorbable type of potassium for the body's cells.

At the end of the day, what we are interested in is that potassium, as efficiently as possible, can do its job of regulating sodium in the body's cells, so the issue of how absorbable one form of potassium is compared to the others is of great importance. There is evidence that potassium citrate may even help reduce bone loss due to osteoporosis.

The potassium supplement dosage that we have recommended for years for each member of the NaturalSlim System is based on their body weight and is as follows:

2 capsules of KADSORB for every 25 pounds (approx. 11 kilograms) of body weight, per day.

For example, a person weighing 150 pounds (68 kilograms) would be using about 12 KADSORB potassium capsules a day. That dose is very safe, if you take into consideration that one large order of french fries from fast-food restaurants contains a total of 862 milligrams of potassium, which would be equivalent to almost 9 capsules of potassium. Unfortunately, the person who eats the order of fries, in addition to the potassium (which is beneficial) also receives an excess of sodium, accompanied by a drastic rise in his glucose produced by the starch in the fries, plus an overdose of fat that is not needed.

When we have cases of people with obesity who also suffer from severe hypertension, we also recommend that they consume two 8-ounce (237 milliliter) glasses of fresh vegetables and leafy green juices every day. That vegetables juice recommendation simply works wonders!

Magnesium MagicMag

The proper functioning of the human body is totally dependent on magnesium because magnesium is essential for more than three hundred different body processes to occur. For example, without magnesium, it becomes impossible to activate the sodium/potassium pump, which is the mechanism that allows cells to remove sodium (salt) from within the cell, while allowing potassium to enter the cell, thus allowing blood pressure to be lowered. Sodium retains water, which increases the body's fluid volume and raises blood pressure, while potassium does the opposite and lowers the pressure. It is magnesium that allows potassium to enter the cells to do its essential job of keeping sodium out.

When a traffic light at an intersection is damaged, and all drivers try to go at the same time, it creates a mess that always results in problems. Sodium (salt) and potassium are like drivers going in different directions, which converge. One could say that magnesium would be the equivalent of a good traffic cop that brings order to the intersection, allowing potassium to enter the cell and sodium to leave the cell. Without magnesium, the tendency of sodium to invade the interior of cells and flood them with water cannot be controlled.

In addition, the pancreas cannot produce insulin and without magnesium, the body's cells lose sensitivity to insulin, thus increasing insulin resistance. Our experience has been that without magnesium neither diabetes nor obesity can be controlled. The basic reason for this is that, if the body's cells are insensitive to insulin (insulin resistance), there is no way to reduce glucose to normal levels.

Magnesium is much more necessary for those with an Excited Nervous System than for those with a Passive Nervous System. But if you suffer from diabetes and especially if you also suffer from hypertension, you need magnesium to control them. We all need magnesium because, without magnesium, insulin cannot be produced efficiently by the pancreas, nor can the body's cells be sensitive to the insulin that your pancreas produces. In other words, to create insulin and for insulin to function at the cellular level, you need to have enough magnesium available to the cells.

There are at least eight different kinds of magnesium (magnesium oxide, magnesium sulfate, etc.), and each has its own characteristics. But we find that the most absorbable form of magnesium is magnesium citrate, in the form of a water-soluble powder. Being a water-soluble powder, magnesium citrate is ingested in its ionic (meaning electrically charged) form, which is the most absorbable form for the body's cells.

Magnesium is called the anti-stress mineral because it is a mineral that relaxes the muscular system and calms the nervous system. Therefore, magnesium supplementation greatly helps people who have difficulty getting good quality sleep. The reason magnesium is so effective in combating constipation is precisely because the intestine is a muscle that relaxes and lets the feces pass once it is supplemented with magnesium. Note, too, that the most important modern medications available to try to control high blood pressure are called "calcium blockers". By blocking the excess calcium that builds up in the walls of the cardiovascular system these medications achieve a relaxation that translates to lower blood pressure and thus control high blood pressure. Magnesium, in its natural form, is the most efficient calcium blocker that the human body has. That is why in many cases lower blood pressure is achieved when the diet is supplemented with sufficient magnesium; especially if it is accompanied by a potassium supplement. Please do not attempt to control your blood pressure or reduce your high blood pressure medications without the help of your physician.

The important point here is that magnesium can be of great help to your metabolism and to your health, especially when combined with a healthy lifestyle, such as the one recommended in this book. Magnesium deficiencies can produce the following:

- agitation, nervousness
- high blood pressure
- anxiety or nervousness
- low body energy
- low stress tolerance or irritability
- difficulty sleeping, insomnia
- headaches, migraines
- backpain due to muscular tension
- muscle spasms and cramps
- constipation
- muscular tension excess
- fatigue or weakness
- fragile bones, osteoporosis
- irritability
- slow metabolism
- uncontrollable glucose levels
- irregular heart rhythm (arrhythmia)
- premenstrual syndrome

Something we noticed at NaturalSlim is that people who supplement their diet with magnesium improve, as they themselves report, their emotional state. This makes quite a bit of sense when we see that there is a study showing that magnesium has a natural antidepressant effect.

One thing that helps is that our MAGICMAG drink, which is prepared by dissolving magnesium citrate powder in cold water or hot water (like a tea), tastes good, which is important. When prepared with 8 ounces (237 milliliters) of hot water, absorption is even better. Our members prepare a hot MAGICMAG magnesium tea at least an hour before bedtime, which allows the body to relax for a good night's sleep. Now, if you have an Excited Nervous System or suffer from hypothyroidism, I recommend that you take MAGICMAG before six o'clock in the evening, so that you can digest it well and it will give you the relaxing effect that helps you sleep. I recommend that you watch Episode #1033 on MetabolismoTV where I explain in detail why it is important to take magnesium at the right time.

People suffering from insomnia or interrupted sleep that causes them to wake up feeling tired, fail to keep their glucose measurements at optimal levels and that does not help them slim down. Sleep quality has a lot to do with your ability to keep your glucose in the normal range and not affect your metabolism.

Dosages for each person's needs vary according to their health condition and accumulated deficiency. One starts with a small dose of one teaspoon daily and gradually increases to three teaspoons or more, depending on your needs. It is important to increase the dose gradually to give the body a chance to incorporate the magnesium into the cells, where it is needed. When the dose is excessive, what occurs is diarrhea due to the relaxing effect that magnesium has on the intestinal system.

The idea is that each person gradually tries different doses until they find the correct dose for their body, which always turns out to be the maximum dose that can be ingested without diarrhea. You may be surprised if your own accumulated magnesium deficiency is so severe that it takes several days of high doses of magnesium before your body signals that you have exceeded the correct maximum dose, causing mild diarrhea.

An example of how to gradually increase the dose of MagicMag magnesium until the correct dose is found would be as follows:

Day	MagicMag dosage used	Observations
Monday	1 teaspoon dissolved in water	I got up two times.
Tuesday	1½ teaspoons dissolved in water	I slept better.
Wednesday	2 teaspoons dissolved in water	I slept better.
Thursday	2½ teaspoons dissolved in water	I slept very well.
Friday	3 teaspoons dissolved in water	I slept well but woke up with diarrhea.
Saturday	I went back to the 2½ teaspoons daily dose, which is my correct dosage	I slept very well and no longer have diarrhea.
Note: You can use hot water (as a tea) or cold water for your daily dose. Your correct dose is the highest dose your body will tolerate, without causing diarrhea. This is called "intestinal tolerance-based dosing".		

The challenge is to find your correct dosage. In the example above, if you were to gradually raise your daily dose to a dose of three teaspoons, and you got diarrhea the next day, that would mean that the three-teaspoon dose exceeded your intestinal tolerance, so your correct dose would be the previous lower dose, which was only 2½ teaspoons a day. You may notice that if you have an excessively stressful day or if you exercise and sweat excessively, your body will tolerate a higher dose of magnesium, because both stress and exercise use up magnesium in the body.

MetabOil 500

Among people suffering from obesity, there are many conditions related to inflammation of the body. Inflammation of the body is a type of warning reaction with which the human body responds to attacks. Wounds, scrapes, burns and traumas experienced by the body's cells always bring with them pain, heat and inflammation that turns the affected area red. Heart problems, autoimmune diseases, arthritis, obesity, insulin resistance and diabetic neuropathy, among others, are all conditions associated with inflammation of the body's tissues.

In metabolic technology, we recognize that any condition that is causing inflammation to the body will prevent it from overcoming obesity. This happens because, in response to inflammation, the body produces its own anti-inflammatory hormone, which is the hormone called cortisol.

Cortisol is a hormone that is produced in the adrenal glands and when an excess of it is produced in response to inflammation, it becomes impossible to slim down, because cortisol, although it has an anti-inflammatory effect, also accumulates fat. The reason why stress is fattening is precisely that, excess cortisol.

For example, a person suffering from a pinched nerve in the back, and who is subject to continuous inflammation and pain, will not be able to simply slim down, because his body will be producing excess cortisol to counteract the inflammation, which will not allow him to reduce body fat.

The same happens when there is severe arthritis, even when there is already a neuropathy in the diabetic patient that maintains a continuous level of pain and inflammation.

All major medications used as anti-inflammatory medications are fattening, because they are primarily based on cortisone[96], which is a hormone that accumulates fat and inhibits the body's ability to reduce fat. This includes the inhalers used by asthmatics, which is why many asthmatics gain weight too easily.

When someone who is taking cortisone-based medications joins the NaturalSlim System, we already know that our metabolism consultants will have to spend a lot of work restoring their metabolism for them to slim down.

One thing we have in our favor is the fact that diets that decrease refined carbohydrates, such as the 3x1 Diet, reduce inflammation in the body in all its manifestations. Therefore, people who come to us with obesity and inflammation, soon

---

[96] cortisone: an anti-inflammatory medication produced by pharmaceutical companies. It is used in injections, tablets, and creams to reduce inflammation. The cortisone medication is virtually identical to the cortisol hormone that our body produces when we face stress and has the effect of making us put on weight.

after they start receiving our help, their inflammation is reduced, which makes it easier for their doctors to decrease the use of anti-inflammatory medications, which otherwise would not allow them to slim down.

However, when we do a candida yeast cleaning in obese people, there can be quite a lot of inflammation since the roots of the fungi are deeply embedded in the tissues. As the yeast is killed by the anti-candida treatment, the roots break off from where they were stuck, leaving small wounds, and causing temporary inflammation, which can be quite severe.

Given this situation of inflammation, which could occur during a candida cleansing, we were looking for a natural supplement to help us reduce inflammation, and we found the so-called evening primrose [97] oil whose scientific name is Gamma-Linolenic Acid or GLA.

Inflammation is significantly reduced when the body is hydrated, and even more so by reducing refined carbohydrates, which are Type F Foods. We needed a natural supplement to help us reduce the inflammation caused by doing the yeast killing (anti-candida) program. We developed the METABOIL 500 supplements composed of GLA oil, to reduce the inflammation and pain that could be caused by the yeast killing and the microscopic wounds left by the dying yeast roots.

Over time, we discovered that METABOIL 500 also served to help reduce inflammation and pain caused by other

---

[97] evening primrose: a plant named *Oenothera biennis* that is cultivated in cold environments such as Canada, from which seeds are extracted from its flower containing the natural oil gamma-linoleic acid or GLA. GLA has an anti-inflammatory and physical pain reducing effect and many clinical studies have been done on it. It is widely used in Europe for inflammatory conditions

conditions such as premenstrual syndrome, arthritis, diabetic neuropathy, and other inflammatory conditions such as multiple sclerosis. In fact, our main interest, was to help reduce inflammation so that the body could reduce its excessive production of the stress hormone cortisol, which would not allow a person to slim down.

METABOIL 500 also increases body temperature for its metabolism boosting effect and helps slim down by restoring the fat burning function of the metabolism, which is why we have used it to help break down stubborn body fat.

Naturally, there is nothing miraculous about this METABOIL GLA oil. The thing is, when you combine different factors that help restore the metabolism, such as good hydration, the 3x1 Diet and intelligently used natural supplements, the results come in no time at all.

As with medications, no natural supplement cures anything; what can be said to be curative is acquiring the knowledge about metabolism to restore it. By getting the correct knowledge and taking responsibility for the condition (diabetes, obesity, or others) your body suffers, it is you who allows your body to recover so that it can function the right way.

Metabolic Protein

To restore metabolism, control diabetes and slim down, you need to understand that breakfast is the most important meal of the day. Your choice of breakfast foods determines, in large part, whether you will spend the rest of your day with erratic (up and down) energy levels, or whether you will enjoy an adequate energy level for the rest of your day. Unstable glucose levels that rise and fall erratically are a product of your dietary food choices, but especially what you eat for breakfast.

Breakfast is called "breakfast" because it is the moment in which "fasting is broken" for about seven to eight hours without having eaten anything, while the body sleeps. If the breakfast is deficient, so will be the rest of the day. The popular saying that "A bad beginning makes a bad ending" is true.

METABOLIC PROTEIN is a high-tech nutritional supplement. It is what they call a meal replacement because it contains all the vitamins and minerals that the FDA (Food and Drug Administration) requires to be called a meal replacement. Common protein shakes (in other countries known as shakes, smoothies, or milk shakes) are not meal replacements because they are not complete foods. A common protein shake or smoothie is a nutritional supplement to enhance the normal diet, but it cannot be used as if it were a complete meal. METABOLIC PROTEIN is a meal replacement; a complete meal that even contains all the vitamins and minerals necessary to sustain the body's metabolism. Usually, we recommend METABOLIC PROTEIN shakes for breakfast only, but they can be used to replace dinner, should you wish to do so.

If some days you decide to also have the shake at night, be sure not to add Coco-10 Plus to your nightly dose, since coconut oil, being a type of saturated fat (the healthy kind), can stimulate your metabolism to the point that it does not allow you to sleep easily. Coco-10 Plus causes a rapid rise in metabolism and provides energy. But you do not want that energy at bedtime because it can take away your sleep. The Coco-10 Plus supplement, which is a liquid oil of which a dose is normally added to Metabolic Protein should be used during the morning or early afternoon hours, but never at night for this very reason.

Whey shakes on the market, besides the fact that they are not meal replacements, have one main problem: they taste bad. This is a real problem because how could you drink a whey protein shake every morning if it becomes a sacrifice to swallow it? We can tell you that you will hardly find a tastier shake than Metabolic Protein. So much so, that it has always been sold at NaturalSlim centers with a satisfaction guaranteed policy, which allows you to return the shake for full credit, if for any reason you do not enjoy its taste, and even if you have already opened the bottle to try it. It took us many years of testing different flavors and finding the most acceptable sweetness levels, but we finally came up with a shake that people enjoy for its taste, even when prepared by mixing the whey protein powder with water only.

Metabolic Protein shakes are low in carbohydrates. Each serving contains only five to seven grams of carbohydrates, so glucose levels rise very little. However, due to their high-absorption whey protein content, these shakes create satiety (a feeling of not being hungry) for five to six hours.

They are available in three flavors: vanilla, chocolate, and strawberry; in Mexico, there are also banana and mocha flavors. Each flavor has its fans. Some people add other flavor touches to the vanilla shake by adding some almond extract or cinnamon powder. You could also add a few strawberries (they are low in fructose). When it comes to flavors, each one is his own master. Flavors are a matter of personal taste. METABOLIC PROTEIN, in surveys we have done, has a level of acceptance of more than 95%. In my book *The Power of Metabolism Recipes*, in addition to delicious meals that will help you slim down, you will find some twenty-five different recipes that you can make with METABOLIC PROTEIN shakes.

Many people with obesity and diabetes have digestive problems (acidity, poor digestion, gases, etc.), which is why we have added powerful enzymes in our METABOLIC PROTEIN shakes that facilitate digestion and increase the absorption of amino acids from whey proteins to about 98%. This allows one dose of METABOLIC PROTEIN to provide an increase in metabolism for long hours. The increased metabolic rate is because almost all (98%) of the amino acids are made readily available to the cells as a source of energy. Common proteins are only absorbed at 70% or less, when not accompanied by special enzymes that increase their absorption.

Each portion of METABOLIC PROTEIN shakes also contain a high dose of the amino acid L-Glutamine. This amino acid controls cravings and eliminates the desire for sweets or sugar. When you make a breakfast with the METABOLIC PROTEIN shake, it is not easy to tempt you with any treats because your glucose and insulin levels remain stable. The amino acid L-Glutamine has a variety of studies showing its health benefits.

The fastest way to increase metabolism and slim down is to use a dose of Coco-10 Plus in your Metabolic Protein shake. This is usually prepared in the morning in a blender or container with a lid that allows you to stir the mixture. Coco-10 Plus does not change the taste of Metabolic Protein. The preparation of the shake that is generally used as a breakfast replacement is as follows:

Formula To Prepare The Metabolic Protein Shake

- 237 milliliters of water (8 ounces)
- Coco-10 Plus tablespoon dosage
- 1 or 2 ice cubes (if you like it colder)
- 2 scoops of Metabolic Protein
- Cinnamon or almond extract to taste

If you want a thicker or thinner consistency, you can increase or decrease the amount of Metabolic Protein powder you use for your shake. For diabetics or people with hypoglycemia, this shake helps maintain normal blood glucose levels, which helps improve both conditions. For other people, what is most noticeable when using this shake for breakfast is that hunger and cravings for sweets or refined carbohydrates disappear.

The combination of Metabolic Protein with Coco-10 Plus has the effect of providing your body with a superior source of energy to boost metabolism. The energy and sense of well-being you feel when using this shake is remarkable. Whey protein extracts have had clinical studies showing several health benefits that may help you, such as lowering blood pressure.

Do not think that this shake will make you slim down on its own. There never have been and never will be any supplements or shakes that are miraculous. No natural nutritional supplement (shakes, smoothies, vitamins capsules or other) alone will achieve anything special for you, if it is not accompanied by lifestyle changes that will improve your metabolism. There are no miracles! Never believe anyone who tries to sell you the idea that some natural supplement cures something or improves something in your metabolism without changing the way you eat or improving your body's hydration.

What really helps you achieve your goals is the metabolism restoration method suggested in this book, which is the same technology we use at NaturalSlim centers.

Metabolic Vitamins

The human body is an amazing organism. It is an entity that always does its best to survive, even despite the harmful actions we constantly inflict on it. However, it is an organism that has basic needs that are vital to its functioning. When these basic needs are denied, the body gradually loses its ability to function well. Slow metabolism or poor metabolism, which in my opinion is causing or aggravating the obesity and diabetes epidemics, is largely caused by vitamins, minerals and micronutrients deficiencies.

A group of prominent researchers from the University of Puerto Rico, who have made important contributions with discoveries on cancer metabolism, accurately described the destructive effects to the metabolism that insufficiencies and deficiencies of vitamins, minerals and micronutrients have. They called their publication *"The Hidden Hunger*

Phenomenon: The Health Impact of Chronic Micronutrient Deficiency or Insufficiency". The "hidden hunger" concept your body's cells have due to a lack of essential vitamins, minerals and micronutrients seemed to me genius and clearly carries the message.

Car engines run on gasoline, oil, and water. Human bodies are far more complex than a car, and the metabolism needs about thirty different types of vitamins and minerals to function. Some of the body's needs are in tiny amounts called micrograms. A microgram is equal to one gram divided by 1,000,000 parts, which is such a small amount that it is impossible to detect without the use of specialized instruments. However, to give an example, if your body needs a certain number of micrograms of the mineral selenium and you do not provide it, your thyroid gland will be affected, and your metabolism will become slow. The thyroid is the gland that controls metabolism, which is why thyroid conditions such as hypothyroidism cause obesity and uncontrolled diabetes. In other words, the lack of a simple nutrient (vitamins, minerals), which weighs less than a hair, will reduce the energy creating capacity of your metabolism and prevent you from slimming down, no matter what you do.

One of the things I discovered when we opened the first NaturalSlim in 1998 was that if there were nutritional insufficiencies or deficiencies in the body of a person with metabolic problems, there was no chance of success. No miracle pill, no exotic herb, no special mineral, or vitamins will overcome a slow metabolism if there are deficiencies of some other vital nutrients.

The vitamins you choose to supplement, their potency and the quality of the nutrients, make a big difference in the results. After an extensive search, I did not find any prefabricated formulation or one that had already been formulated by any vitamins manufacturer that would really allow us to be satisfied. Therefore, I had to create a high potency formulation that also took into consideration the following seven goals:

1. Doses of the important **B-Complex** (B1, B2, B3, etc.) need to be no less than 50 milligrams of each, thus activating the metabolism. The entire B-Complex group of vitamins is vital for metabolism.

2. Must have **all the minerals** plus **micronutrients** that activate the body's enzymes that dominate the hormonal system, to help restore metabolism.

3. They should contain the maximum doses allowed of fat-soluble vitamins, such as **Vitamins A and D**, which are used to protect eyesight, to improve calcium absorption and to boost the immune system.

4. The content of **Vitamin E** should be in its natural form (not synthetic), since it has been demonstrated that it performs its vital function of protecting the body better.

5. You need a dose of **Vitamin C** that really covers the needs.

6. You must help the body to **detoxify** so it needs the help of compounds such as MSM (methylsulfonylmethane) which is a natural source of sulfur.

7. People with slow metabolism do not digest well. It must contain **digestive enzymes** to be able to absorb vitamins and minerals well.

When I took all these above requirements to vitamins manufacturers, several treated me like a weirdo. They could not understand that I was demanding so many different nutrients, in such high doses, and of a quality that was obviously more expensive. In reality, I was trying to provide a person's body's metabolism with everything it needed. I wanted to guarantee good results, because I knew that even the lack of a micronutrient of which very small doses are used could sabotage the restoration of the metabolism.

In general, people who come to NaturalSlim centers have already tried everything and failed multiple diet plans, simply because they never had the opportunity to learn how to restore their body's metabolism. Failing them by saving a few dollars by acquiring a deficient vitamin supplement was not an option.

Adequate vitamins, minerals and micronutrients are an important factor in helping to restore the metabolism. Many years of consuming processed foods, fried foods, sugar and refined carbohydrates, combined with consuming too little vegetables and salad, take their toll on the body and are reflected in deficiencies that weaken the metabolism. Metabolism can be restored when the correct things are done to achieve it. Restoring the energy-generating capacity of the metabolism can control diabetes, obesity and a number of other health conditions.

The METABOLIC VITAMINS formula is, to my knowledge, the most complete I have seen. It is true that they are a few packets of daily dose that bring a combination of several tablets or capsules that may seem like a lot. People who use these vitamins formula to boost their metabolism consume a complete packet every day. This metabolism boosting vitamins formula should be taken with food and never on an empty stomach, because these compounds, although natural, are concentrated and should be taken with food. Some people complain that "there are so many pills to take every day", but once they start to see that their clothes fit bigger and their energy level has greatly increased, they stop complaining. Nothing speaks as clearly as the results!

PassivOil

After the fundamental discovery that it is indeed the Central Nervous System that directs everything that happens in our body's metabolism, I pursued deeper and deeper into the scope of the devastating effects that could be caused by an overly Excited Nervous System.

To my horror I discovered that the scientific literature reveals that behind every cancer condition there is an over Excited Nervous System. The same thing happens behind every autoimmune condition where the body seems to attack itself as if the Central Nervous System has been hijacked by a psychotic madman.

Realizing the vital importance of discovering effective ways to activate the Passive Nervous System to counteract the devastating effect of an over Excited Nervous System, I explored all fields related to metabolism and health. Sometime later I discovered the fascinating world of essential oils.

Essential oils are highly concentrated versions of natural plant oils. These oils are produced using distillation processes that yield a highly concentrated oil and many of them have therapeutic or healing properties.

I was especially interested in finding out which oils had proven calming effects on the Excited Nervous System, or the opposite, which was to know which essential oils had effects that reinforced the activity of the Passive Nervous System.

I discovered that essential oils, when they are of real purity and potency, can almost instantly reverse a crisis of over-stimulation of the Excited Nervous System. It turns out that essential oils work by acting through the olfactory system or by being absorbed by the skin. I discovered in the scientific literature evidence of how a certain essential oil was able to stop the growth of cancer in the brain, for which traditional medicine had no solution.

Essential oils, or aromatic oils as they were called in ancient times, have been used by many cultures throughout the world for many centuries. The uses of essential oils have ranged from ceremonial religious purposes, such as the use of incense, to healing the sick.

I spent a lot of time researching the subject of essential oils and thoroughly examining the scientific evidence behind these oils. I started recommending them to people who had serious conditions, tumors, or cancer, because I saw a lot of hope in finding some way to activate the Passive Nervous System, which is the one that heals the body or calms the Excited Nervous System, which I could say is the one that destroys the body when it is overexcited.

I did hundreds of tests with my metabolism consultants who served as guinea pigs for my experiments with essential oils. I included at times some members of the NaturalSlim System who were experiencing severe insomnia, states of severe anxiety, cancerous tumors, or autoimmune disease with the idea of helping them to activate the Passive Nervous System and at the same time, to test the calming results that the various essential oils could have.

In fact, I discovered that essential oils could be a wonderful tool to quickly calm the nervous system and with them achieve improvements in metabolism and health.

With the idea of creating a blend of essential oils that would be calming to the nervous system, I continued digging deeper into the subject of essential oils and began to discover manufacturers and sellers of essential oils selling at unrealistically low prices, while a few others were selling the same essential oil, from the same plant, at very high prices. Such drastically different price differences made no sense.

Exploring this topic further, I realized that the internet and online stores, such as Amazon.com, were cluttered with fake essential oils and oils mixed with synthetic pollutants. True essential oils, when pure and of high potency, are expensive like everything else that is scarce. I observed hundreds of illogical offers such as, for example, an offer for a 120 milliliter (4 ounce) bottle of the popular lavender essential oil, which claimed to be pure and of therapeutic (healing) quality and was being sold on Amazon for only $15.95 retail. However, a distiller manufacturer that extracted lavender oil in Greece, directly from the plants, had a factory cost equivalent to $45.00 in the same size bottle. So, Amazon's supplier of this lavender essential oil offered the supposed "pure oil" for only ⅓ of the cost at the factory that distilled it in large quantities.

I finally bought several samples on Amazon of the essential oils they were selling at ridiculously cheap prices, like $15.95, and sent them to Dr. Robert Pappas of Essential Oil University. Essential Oil University is an organization that does laboratory testing of essential oils to expose those unscrupulous merchants who gamble with the public's health by selling them fraudulent oils full of synthetic chemicals. I discovered that all the oils being offered at very cheap prices were fraudulent. Dr. Pappas supplied me with laboratory tests showing that over 80% of the essential oils offered on the internet are fraudulent.

After this eye-opening experience of discovering that the essential oil business is plagued by fraud and adulteration and knowing that essential oils really did work to calm the Excited Nervous System, I spent several months locating distilling factories that were willing to provide us with samples of their oils to test their purity with Dr. Pappas' laboratories.

We wanted to combine essential oils of high purity to prepare a harmonious blend of essential oils that we would call PASSIVOIL or oils to activate the Passive Nervous System.

PASSIVOIL is a blend of three essential oils of guaranteed purity that our members of the NaturalSlim System or anyone else can use confidently with their family and even with their children, when they want to help them calm the Excited Nervous System.

High potency essential oils should not be used completely pure on the skin because they can cause irritation, which is why PASSIVOIL is a dilution in coconut oil. Coconut oil is an oil that quickly penetrates the skin and therefore helps to transport the essential oil blend safely into the body. It is not recommended to ingest these oils as ingestion can be dangerous. PASSIVOIL is used either as a topical rub on the skin or to inhale its essences, which is the quickest way to bring the relaxing and calming effect to the Central Nervous System.

PASSIVOIL can bring calm and relaxation to an overly Excited Nervous System and that is a great help in achieving good results with the metabolism of a person going through a health crisis.

RELAXSLIM SUPPLEMENT WITH ADAPTOGENS

A few years ago I had the pleasure to personally meet a Russian scientist, who influenced my thinking about metabolism. This scientist, Dr. Zakir Ramazanov, was a Russian professor, specialized in plant biochemistry and molecular biology. He had thoroughly studied the properties of different extracts of plants, herbs, and algae.

Dr. Ramazanov wrote and published hundreds of scientific articles and several books about adaptogens and algae. Zakir Ramazanov had several approved patents in the field of biotechnology, plant biochemistry, molecular biology, and various active plant compounds.

Dr. Ramazanov was a professor at the Technological Institute, at the University of Madrid in Spain, at Louisiana State University (USA) and a Senior Scientist of the Russian Academy of Sciences. His achievements include being recognized for his work in growing natural organisms on the Russian space station MIR.

During the time of the so-called "cold war" between Russia and the United States, Dr. Ramazanov worked for more than ten years researching the properties of adaptogens for the Russian Academy of Sciences. That was a time when the Russians were interested in knowing and mastering the metabolic energizing properties of adaptogens, with the idea of gaining an advantage over their main adversaries, the United States of America, at the Olympic and military levels. Practically all the research done by the Russians on adaptogens was done secretly for these reasons.

With the help of Dr. Ramazanov, who had already emigrated to the United States, and with whom I became good friends, we created a supplement we call RelaxSlim, which contains a combination of twenty-one different natural compounds that have been shown to improve metabolism. They are natural substances that reduce the effects of stress, reduce the growth of candida albicans yeast, provide support for the thyroid gland, which is vital for improving metabolism.

RelaxSlim comes in capsules and only two capsules are used at breakfast and two capsules at lunch. We identified natural substances with guaranteed higher potency of the active compounds to avoid having to use dozens of capsules per day with lower potency.

RelaxSlim contains the vitamins and minerals that prevent the candida albicans yeast from continuing to grow and spread uncontrollably inside the body, which is one of the problems of diabetics. They are natural supplements such as biotin, which is a B Complex vitamin. This vitamin stops the reproductive system of the candida yeast and controls its growth. In addition, biotin has been shown to help reduce glucose levels in diabetics.

We also use a relatively high dose of niacin (Vitamin B3) in this supplement. Niacin is a fungicidal vitamin, that is, it kills fungi. It also has an antidepressant effect. None of this is true of niacinamide, which is the type of Vitamin B3 used by most vitamin manufacturers.

Commercial vitamin manufacturers substitute niacin (Vitamin B3), which is a vitamin in its natural state of multiple benefits to the metabolism, for niacinamide which is an industry creation to prevent niacin from causing a reaction when it hits toxins or fungi in the body.

Niacin is a detoxifying agent, which is why it can cause reddening of the skin in people whose bodies are full of toxins. For example, when in 1986 there was the nuclear accident in Chernobyl, Russia, high doses of niacin (Vitamin B3) were given to the population to help them extract the accumulated radiation in their bodies.

If you start using RelaxSlim and notice that the skin on your face becomes very red at times, you are not in any danger. Only your body is being cleansed of accumulated toxins and in some time you will stop having these reactions.

RelaxSlim contains herbs such as guggul and the adaptogen ashwagandha, which support the thyroid gland. It also contains all the vitamins and minerals that are essential for the body and thyroid to convert the T4 hormone produced by the thyroid into the T3 hormone, which is the hormone that speeds up metabolism. It contains a natural compound called "myricetin" which has been shown in controlled studies that it increases the absorption of the mineral iodine by the thyroid. Iodine is essential to produce thyroid hormones.

The RelaxSlim supplement has another benefit in that it contains the adaptogen rhodiola rosea, which has a natural anti-stress, antidepressant, and energizing effect. This adaptogen, rhodiola rosea, also has the effect of increasing sexual potency and appetite in both men and women. For this reason, it has been used in Russia as an aphrodisiac for many generations. In Russia there has been a custom of giving a small jar of rhodiola rosea to newly married couples to ensure the couple's fertility.

RelaxSlim also contains other adaptogens such as rhaponticum carthamoides (leuza) and rhododendron caucasicum, which increase cellular energy throughout the body, including improving intellectual and learning capacity.

The RelaxSlim supplement has been one of our most effective tools to help restore the metabolism of people with obesity and people with diabetes. We really like the fact that this supplement does not affect the nervous system, because it does not contain any stimulating agents. In fact, we called it RelaxSlim because we noticed that by improving cellular metabolism and increasing cellular energy, it was able to help people slim down, but while maintaining a "relaxed" state, which is ideal.

Especially for people with hypothyroidism, who suffer from a slow metabolism that makes it difficult for them to slim down, and for diabetics whose energy levels are often not the best, using RelaxSlim makes a noticeable difference.

While this supplement can help you by supporting your body's natural metabolic processes, it should be clear that **it is not a drug** and is not intended to cure or treat any disease or condition. Only physicians are qualified to treat conditions such as diabetes and associated diseases.

Restoring metabolism has everything to do with improving your body's **energy** production. In that sense, the RelaxSlim supplement can be a good aid in combination with metabolism restoration techniques.

Stress Defender For Stress

Through many years of working with people suffering from a slow metabolism, we realized that stress is one of the biggest enemies of the metabolism. To restore the metabolism, it is necessary to control the harmful effects of stress.

Many of us live a life full of stressful situations that sometimes last for too long. In fact, stress can be so continuous and habitual that we consider it normal, when in fact stress is anything but normal. Financial problems, family problems, stressful work environments, plus a host of other bad news that hits us daily, force our bodies to produce the cortisol stress hormone.

The cortisol hormone creates a hormonal conflict in the body because it interferes with the hormones produced in the thyroid gland, which reduces our metabolism and creates a tendency to accumulate more fat. Cortisol also causes the body to react with drastic rises and falls in blood glucose levels, which will not allow you to slim down or properly control glucose levels. Even when cortisol levels in the blood are very high, we may begin to suffer from insomnia or difficulty sleeping.

People who experience a lot of stress usually sleep poorly or wake up tired in the morning. Stress triggers the production of cortisol, and this causes havoc both with the hormonal system and the body's nervous system.

Stress kills people. But before it kills them, it makes most of them put on weight, because it reduces their metabolism and accumulates fat, especially in the abdominal area (belly). To control diabetes or slim down, it is necessary to be as free as possible from the effects of stress and not to be suffering from anxiety. There are also people whose states of anxiety cause them to eat sweets or refined carbohydrates, and if they do not control their anxiety, they will not be able to improve their metabolism either.

Over more than twenty years, as I have helped thousands of people restore their metabolism and slim down, I have seen the negative effects of stressful situations. Even having to take care of a couple of undisciplined children can send your cortisol levels through the roof, so much so that your glucose levels go out of control, you put on weight, or prevent you from slimming down.

The stress management supplement we created is called STRESS DEFENDER. It is a very effective natural supplement that controls the negative effects of stress by making the body produce much less cortisol. We have had dozens of grateful wives and husbands come to thank us for the calming and anti-stress effect this supplement has had on their partner.

The STRESS DEFENDER supplement in combination with MAGICMAG magnesium, has been our best natural solution for those people who are unable to get a good night's sleep, because they suffer from insomnia, wakefulness or have a too much interrupted sleep. We already know, from experience, that if a person does not have a good quality of sleep, they will not be able to control their glucose levels and it will be practically impossible for them to slim down. To restore metabolism and to control diabetes, stress must be controlled and that also includes improving the quality of sleep.

TESTOSTERIN

All organs, glands, tissues, muscles, nerves and bones in the body are controlled by hormones. Hormones in turn are very powerful substances that can give orders to the cells of the body and therefore can modify the structure of the body.

Many of us have heard of athletes and baseball players who have injected hormones to gain greater physical strength and endurance. Several well-known athletes have been tempted by so-called anabolics (muscle building hormones). The temptation is great because when a person injects an anabolic his muscles grow and strengthen, and this achieves a superior athletic performance that provides him with an unmatched competitive advantage. Although it is an illegal and immoral way to compete against other athletes, the temptation is great because every athlete wants to be the best in his sport.

In the field of natural supplements there are certain substances that help improve women's hormonal system and others that help men's hormonal system.

Women who want to slim down use the natural progesterone cream to minimize the effects of estrogen which is a female hormone that makes them fat. But, until now we had nothing to help the hormonal system of men who want to slim down.

We were doing research and discovered that the hormonal system of men could be improved by naturally increasing the production of the male testosterone hormone. Scientific studies show that after the age of 30, men gradually lose part of their testosterone production. For example, it is estimated that at the age of 50, a man's body produces approximately 50% of the amount of testosterone it produced when he was young. By age 60 it is reduced to 40% and by age 70 testosterone production can be as low as 20% of what it was originally.

It is known that the testosterone hormone is the one that creates strong muscles and contributes to a well-defined body. This is the reason why as men get older their bodies start to become flabbier, with less muscle and more fat. Testosterone is a hormone that, when building large and strong muscles in a man's body, it also contributes to reduce body fat because, of the body's tissues, the muscles are the ones that consume the most body fat.

When a man does resistance exercises such as weightlifting his body builds muscle and this creates an increase in muscle mass. Muscle in turn consumes body fat and creates a lean, well-defined body. If a man manages to increase his natural testosterone production, he will also achieve a substantial increase in muscle mass and a reduction in body fat. As a man's testosterone production rises, he may not lose weight because the new muscles weigh two and a half times more than the fat, but his body will get leaner, and he will have energy to spare.

The other benefit of increasing a man's natural testosterone production is that it can have a very positive effect on his health and sexual performance. Testosterone is the hormone that maintains sexual interest towards a partner and contributes to the frequency and healthy enjoyment of sexual activity in couples. There are even studies that show that men with higher testosterone levels have far fewer cardiovascular incidents.

We created a product called TESTOSTERIN with the purpose of offering hormonal help to men. This product contains an extract of natural origin called testosfen which in clinical studies demonstrated an increase of up to 98% in the production of testosterone in men. TESTOSTERIN contains several ingredients aimed at creating increased testosterone production and several antioxidants that are used to protect the body's production of nitric oxide. Nitric oxide is the molecule that allows men to have a satisfactory erection and was the discovery that led to the creation of the Viagra medication.

TESTOSTERIN, in addition to increasing testosterone production, achieves an increase in nitric oxide production. This increase in nitric oxide not only is good for men's sexual activity and health, but it also has the effect of relaxing the cardiovascular system and, in people with high blood pressure, can help normalize it by naturally relaxing the tension in the arteries.

It is worth mentioning that men who are sexually active have a better disposition to maintain their weight and figure. In the matter of improving metabolism and slim down, the emotional state and the general attitude of the person towards life are determining factors. Healthy partner sex fosters a sense of affinity between the couple and is an excellent way to get rid of stress. As we know, stress produces another hormone called cortisol that makes us fat, and that is why healthy sexual activity can help both men and women to slim down without so much effort.

There are several studies that show that among diabetic men, testosterone levels are significantly lower than among men without diabetes. One of the most disastrous consequences of diabetes is that it often leads to impotence in men. TESTOSTERONE can be a great help for men, especially if the man is over 30 years old or if he suffers from diabetes or high blood pressure.

GLOSSARY:
DEFINITIONS OF WORDS AND TERMS

3x1 Diet: a dietary regimen for metabolism restoration that considers the different effects that each type of food can have on the body's hormonal system (e.g., the amount of insulin the pancreas needs to produce). In addition, the 3x1 Diet is individually adapted for each person considering their biological individuality and the reaction that their CENTRAL Nervous System will have according to whether their nervous system is predominantly PASSIVE or EXCITED. A special feature is that in the 3x1 Diet foods are categorized as Type S Foods (SLIMMING – Helps SUPPORT the control of diabetes)or Type F Foods (FATTENING – Act as a FOE (ENEMIES) for the control of diabetes). The 3x1 Diet® is a registered trademark by Frank Suárez in the United States, Mexico and other countries in Latin America and Europe.

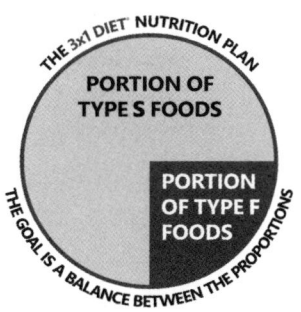

acetaminophen: acetaminophen, also known in other countries as paracetamol, is a widely used analgesic. Analgesic means pain reliever and is used for headaches, muscle aches, fever, sinus infections and sore throat. It is sold under different brand names such as Tylenol, Panadol, Mapap, Ofrimev, Feverall, and Acephen, among others. In addition to these products, acetaminophen is contained in more than six hundred other products as part of the formulation of many, many other medications.

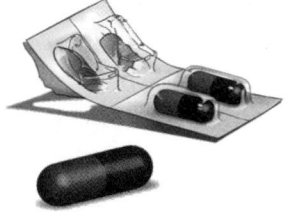

acidity or alkalinity: it is measured on the "pH" scale, which stands for "potential of hydrogen". The more hydrogen a substance contains, the more acid it is, the less hydrogen it contains, the more alkaline it is. Observe the below pH scale of different common substances.

SUBSTANCES	pH VALUE	ALKALINE / ACID
ammonia (Clorox or other brands)	11.9	ALKALINE
milk of magnesia	10.5	ALKALINE
toothpaste	9.9	ALKALINE
baking soda	8.4	ALKALINE
human blood	7.4	ALKALINE
pure water	7.0	NEUTRAL
human urine	6.0	ACID
tequila	5.2	ACID
black coffee	5.0	ACID
beer	4.5	ACID
wine	3.5	ACID
vinegar	2.9	ACID
soft drinks (coke & others)	2.5	ACID
digestion gastric juices	2.0	ACID

adrenals: above each of our two kidneys we have a gland that produces the adrenaline hormone which is a stress hormone. For this reason, they are called the adrenal glands. The adrenals also produce other hormones, mainly the cortisol hormone which, among other things, accumulates fat in the body and is the reason why stress is fattening.

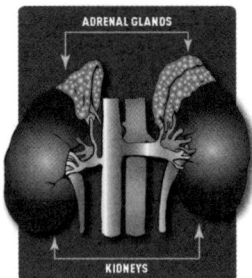

GLOSSARY: DEFINITIONS OF WORDS AND TERMS

allergies: an allergy is a specific response of the immune system, which is the defense system in our body. It is a specific reaction to certain foods or substances that develops an immediate reaction such as itching, mucus, headache, or other manifestations.

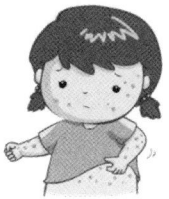

amino acids: amino acids are the tiny components that make up proteins (meats, seafoods, cheeses, eggs, etc.). Depending on the types of amino acids in a protein is that you can differentiate between different types of proteins, such as between types of meats: pork, chicken, turkey, fish, etc.

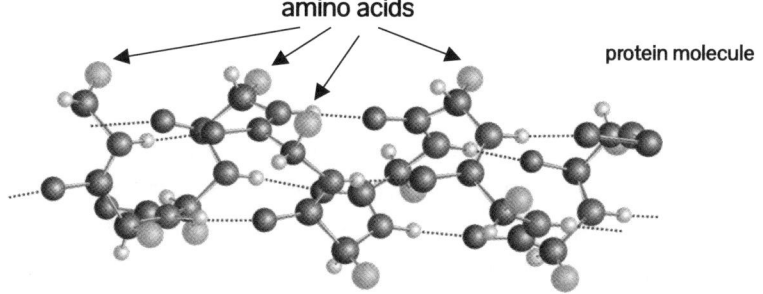

ammonia: is a substance consisting of a gas dissolved in water, which has a strong odor and is widely used in cleaning supplies. One of its most common uses is to clean glass, porcelain, and stainless steel; it is sold as a detergent.

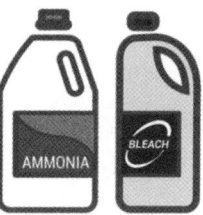

arteries: these are the vessels or passages through which blood leaves the heart and reaches all parts of the body. They are the equivalent of what would be the body's pipeline through which the blood circulates.

arthritis: the word arthritis is composed of "-itis" meaning inflammation and "arthros" meaning joint, which is a place where one bone meets another. Inflammation of the bone joints is called arthritis.

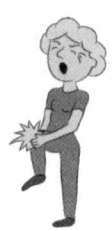

atherosclerosis: a condition in which the walls of the body's arteries (heart, brain, etc.) become inflamed, suffer damage and fill with a plaque of fat and calcium that clogs circulation. Arteriosclerosis or atherosclerosis hardens and stiffens the arteries, so they lose the flexibility to expand when the heart pumps and blood pressure (tension) rises. Arteries also become blocked and that is what causes a heart attack or a stroke.

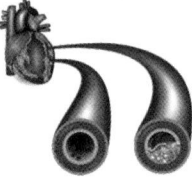

clogged artery

atoms: the atom is the smallest unit particle of matter or substance that can exist. Solid matter, food and substances are all composed of atoms that form them when they are joined together. The word atom comes from Greek and means "not divisible".

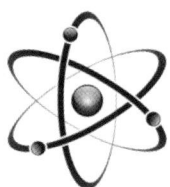

ATP: the term ATP stands for "adenosine triphosphate". ATP is a type of chemical energy that is created when the body's cells, within the mitochondria, efficiently convert the food we eat into energy with the help of oxygen. If a person's body were to produce a greater amount of ATP in the cells, the person would feel that they have strength and an abundance of energy as their metabolism would be boosted as well as their ability to slim down.

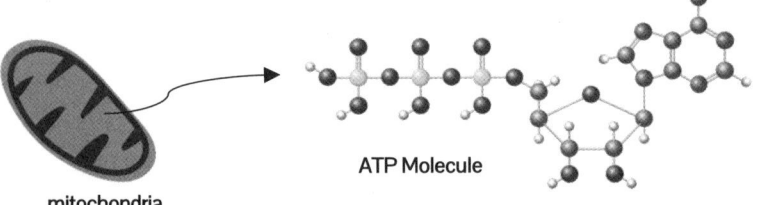

mitochondria   ATP Molecule

GLOSSARY: DEFINITIONS OF WORDS AND TERMS

autoimmune: refers to a disease in which the body's defense system, which is the immune system, attacks and destroys its own cells. The cause of autoimmune diseases is unknown, but everything indicates that the body has suffered some extreme incident, which is stressful and has caused some intolerance, or there is some toxic, food or substance, or some virus that attacks it, which creates a state of confusion in the immune system, where it attacks itself, as if it were its own enemy.

AUTONOMOUS Nervous System: is the part of the nervous system that controls the body's involuntary actions (that you do not have to think about). The AUTONOMOUS Nervous System controls the heart, lungs, pancreas, liver, intestine, and all the body's vital hormonal processes. It is what causes the heart rate to accelerate automatically when someone is frightened, the blood pressure to rise, or the blood glucose to rise in a diabetic, even if he or she has not eaten. It is called AUTONOMOUS because it cannot be controlled by the mind; it operates independently of a person's thoughts.

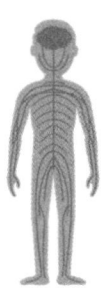

biological individuality: differences between the bodies of different people due to hereditary factors that affect everything in the body, including blood type.

brain: is the part of the nervous system where our thoughts, perceptions (seeing, smelling, tasting, hearing) and emotions cause changes in all the functions of all the other parts of the body. The brain also generates the electrical impulses that control involuntary movements, or autonomous movements, such as breathing, heart rate, digestion, and others.

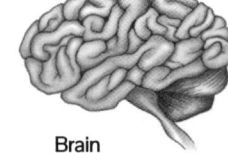

Brain

calories: the term calorie comes from French, which in turn originated from Latin "calor". In fact, a calorie is a measure of heat. It was a term created by French professor Nicholas Clément around 1819, to describe and calculate the conversion of the energy contained in coal when burned inside a boiler, to heat water to the point of converting it into steam to move a train engine. Although the term calorie originated in the physics of steam engines, the American chemist Wilbur Olin Atwater found and used it for the first time in 1875 in connection with his 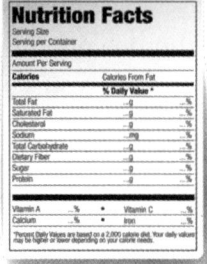 studies on nutrition and human metabolism. Atwater was the first to create the tables of nutritional values of foods and since then the term calorie went from measuring the energy of a steam boiler to measuring the energy that a food could supply to the human body.

candida albicans yeast: candida albicans is one of more than 150 species of yeast that inhabit the human body. It is so called because this yeast is white in color. The word *candida* comes from the Latin word *candidus* which means bright white; and the word *albicans* comes from the Latin word *albus* which also means white. All human beings have candida albicans yeast in our body and, under normal conditions, this yeast does not invade or cause disease. But if you neglect your nutrition by consuming an excess of refined carbohydrates, which is its favorite food, the candida yeast will reproduce aggressively in all parts of your body. This yeast produces 78 different toxics that create a slow metabolism and an impressive variety of diseases. Cancer patients, people with weak constitution, people with obesity and people with diabetes have, for the most part, bodies that are severely infected with candida albicans yeast.

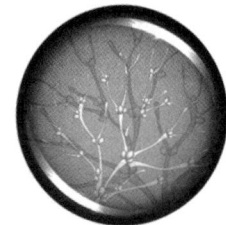
Candida Albicans Yeast

carbohydrates: carbohydrates cover a wide variety of foods such as bread, flour, pizza, tortillas, rice, potatoes, grains, sweets, sugar, and include vegetables (greens) and salads. When we say "refined carbohydrates" we refer to those carbohydrates that have been processed, cooked, ground, polished or refined in some way, making them much more absorbable and easily raising the body's glucose levels. Almost all vegetables and salads (except for corn) are considered "natural carbohydrates" (unrefined).

cardiac palpitations: if your heart rate is too fast (more than 100 beats per minute), it is called tachycardia, if it is too slow it is called bradycardia, and if it is irregular, it is called arrhythmia. Any abnormal rhythm condition is cause for concern.

cells: cells are the smallest parts of the body that contain life. In fact, cells, although extremely small, feed, digest and breathe just like you do. The health of your body depends on the health of the cells in your body.

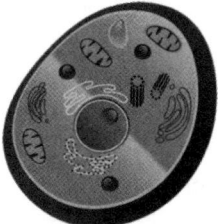
Animal Cell

cholesterol: cholesterol is a natural substance produced by the human body and by animals. Cholesterol is the main building material of many hormones, such as the estrogen hormone, which is the female hormone, and the testosterone hormone, which is the male hormone. All cells in the body contain cholesterol, except for the bone cells.

circadian cycle: the word circadian comes from the Latin word *circa* which means "around" and from the Latin word *dies* which means "day". So, the circadian cycle refers to the changes that occur to living beings at regular time intervals and that are repeated daily.

clinical studies: clinical studies are publications of scientific studies that have been carried out by physicians and scientific researchers from universities and gather scientific evidence on a subject related to medicine or health.

combustion: energy-creating reaction of a fuel with oxygen.

combustion

cortisol: is a natural anti-inflammatory hormone produced by the human body in the adrenal glands. Cortisol is produced in the body under stressful conditions. It has an anti-inflammatory effect, but also increases body fat levels especially in the abdominal area.

cortisone: an anti-inflammatory medication produced by pharmaceutical companies. It is used in injections, tablets, and creams to reduce inflammation. The medication cortisone is virtually identical to the cortisol hormone that our body produces when we face stress and has the effect of making us put on weight.

cycle: a series of phases, states or actions that occur one after the other and, at the end of the sequence, occur again in the same order. Some examples are the menstrual cycle, the solar cycle, the cycle of the seasons.

GLOSSARY: DEFINITIONS OF WORDS AND TERMS

debug: to cleanse or purify.

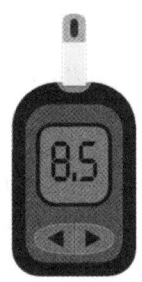

diabetes: diabetes is a condition characterized by having glucose (blood sugar) levels that are excessively high and harmful to the body's health.

diabetic neuropathy: a type of nerve damage that occurs in people who have diabetes. This damage makes it difficult for the nerves to carry messages to the brain and other parts of the body. A diabetic may lose sensation in his or her legs to the point that he or she cannot feel the pain of a steel nail being driven into the heel of a leg. Diabetic neuropathy is also the cause of loss of sexual potency in diabetic men and the cause of sexual frigidity in diabetic women. Amputations usually occur after the person has already begun to experience some degree of diabetic neuropathy.

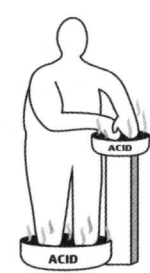
DIABETIC NEUROPATHY

diagnostics: the word diagnostic is formed from *diag-* which means "through" and *gnosis* which means "knowledge". A diagnostic is a decision that a physician or health professional makes based on his knowledge of the condition or disease and what he observes in the patient.

digestion: is the natural process that allows the body to transform food into nutrients that can be used for the creation of energy produced by metabolism.

Digestive System

diuretic: a medication that works by extracting and reducing the volume of water in the human body to reduce blood pressure.

When a diuretic is used, the person increases the volume of urine excretion and thus reduces the pressure.

diverticulum: is a pouch that forms in the wall of the intestine. When they become inflamed, they can produce several unpleasant and painful symptoms, known as. diverticulitis.

enzyme: enzymes are proteins that participate in achieving changes and transformations of other substances. For example, there is an enzyme that transforms cholesterol and converts it into the estrogen hormone. There are different enzymes that are used to digest fats, proteins, and carbohydrates. There are enzymes involved in all processes in the body.

excited: this name proved to be very effective so that the people that we were helping with the metabolism could learn it, associate it, and remember it, although I had to clarify to my friends from Mexico that "excited" has nothing to do with sexuality, since in their country "excited" has a sexual connotation.

fiber: is one of the components of carbohydrates. Although it is considered part of carbohydrates, it is a part that does not increase glucose and cannot make you fat. In fact, fiber helps reduce glucose absorption, thus helping you slim down. You could say that fiber is like a grain and does not provide any nutritional value, nor does it affect glucose.

fixed idea: a decision or thought about something, which is unchangeable.

GLOSSARY: DEFINITIONS OF WORDS AND TERMS

flora: a collection of organisms such as bacteria, some viruses, parasites, and fungi that live inside the body on the walls of the intestine and the vagina in women. Most of these organisms help in different body processes and are harmless. However, some of them, under specific conditions, can cause damage to the body, such as, for example, the overgrowth of the candida yeast, which can invade the whole body and cause damage when a person consumes an excess of refined carbohydrates.

fuel: any material (gasoline, coal, etc.) capable of releasing energy when oxidized (it bonds with oxygen.

genes: genes are microscopic markers that all body cells contain and serve to determine the traits that a living organism (person, plant, yeast, bacteria, etc.) will inherit because they transmit hereditary factors from one generation to the next. If, for example, mom and dad had green eyes there would be a strong possibility that a child of theirs would inherit the trait of green eyes. Genes transmit traits from parents to their children. Plants also have genes that pass on their characteristics and traits to their offspring.

genetically modified: a genetically modified organism (abbreviated GMO) is a plant, animal, yeast, or bacteria to which certain genes† have been added by genetic engineering to produce certain traits or characteristics. In the case of corn, it is a corn plant whose genetic material has been artificially altered using genetic engineering techniques.

gland: is a body organ that has the capacity to produce substances that produce effects in other parts of the body.

Thyroid Gland

glucagon: a hormone produced by the pancreas that has the effect of reducing hunger and helps burn stored body fat (obesity), thus having the opposite effect of insulin, which is a hormone that causes hunger and accumulates fat.

glucose: blood sugar that is the fuel and main nutrient of the body's cells.

glycogen: a type of starch (imagine mashed potatoes) that the liver creates naturally to store glucose. This allows it to keep blood glucose levels stable between meals. Glycogen is like a fuel reserve that is stored in the liver and muscles until the body needs it to increase blood glucose levels.

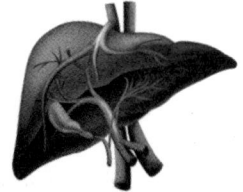
The Liver

goitrogens: are natural or chemical substances that have been demonstrated to suppress the function of the thyroid gland. Anything that suppresses thyroid gland function reduces metabolism. Some natural goitrogens are contained in soy. The fluoride in toothpaste is also a goitrogen that reduces thyroid hormone production.

gout: gout is a disease caused by an accumulation of uric acid crystals in different parts of the body, especially in the big toes, soft tissues, and kidneys. It is a type of arthritis attack that causes intense pain and redness that is especially aggravated at night.

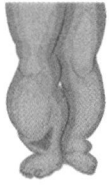

helicobacter pylori bacteria: bacteria that lives exclusively in the human stomach. It is a spiral bacterium (its shape resembles the blades of a helicopter) which is why it acquired its name "helicobacter". Indeed, its spiral shape allows it to penetrate and screw itself into the stomach wall, which is why it is accused of being the cause of stomach ulcers.

homeostasis: is a compound word from the Greek homo meaning similar and stasis meaning state or stability. Homeostasis is a property of living organisms that consists of their ability to maintain a stable internal condition, using metabolism to compensate for changes in their environment (food, temperature, hydration, etc.). It is a form of dynamic equilibrium, made possible by a network of control systems in the human body.

hormones: hormones are messenger substances in the body that carry commands that cause changes in the body. For example, the female hormone communicates messages to the body's cells that create feminine features (with breasts, no beard, more fat, and less muscles), while the male testosterone hormone carries the opposite message of creating male bodies (no breasts, beard, less fat and more muscle).

hydrochloric acid: acid produced by the stomach to help digest food.

hypertension: excessively high blood pressure. High blood pressure increases the likelihood of suffering a cerebrovascular accident, heart attack, heart failure, kidney disease or premature death.

hyperthyroidism: is a condition in which the thyroid gland produces an excess of thyroid hormones. This causes weight loss, palpitations, high blood pressure, insomnia, and panic attacks among others.

hypochlorhydria: a condition in which the stomach has a deficient production of hydrochloric acid (HCL), which causes indigestion that develops into stomach acidity. The manifestations are almost identical to those of gastroesophageal reflux for which several other medications are also promoted.

hypoglycemia: is an abnormal reduction in blood glucose levels, which can cause dizziness, headache, cold sweats, mental disorientation and even unconsciousness. In principle, the body's cells begin to die from starvation due to the lack of glucose, some die, and the nervous and hormonal systems go out of control. This occurs when the blood glucose drops too low (below 60 ml/dl), which can happen due to an overdose of insulin, going too many hours without eating or intolerance reactions to certain carbohydrates such as rice or sugar.

hypothermia: means that the body temperature is too low, as would be experienced by someone suffering from the crushing cold of the North Pole, from which they may die. It also happens to shipwrecked survivors who are forced to float for a long time in seas where the water temperature is too cold.

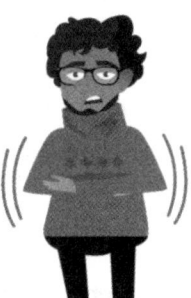

hypothyroidism: a condition in which the thyroid gland produces an insufficient amount of the hormones that control metabolism, body temperature and body energy. This condition is characterized by symptoms such as depression, hair loss, cold extremities, constipation, dry skin, difficulty losing weight, continuous fatigue, digestive problems and continuous infections. It is a condition that is not always detected in laboratory tests and may exist sub-clinically (not easily detected in laboratory tests).

insulin: a very important hormone produced in the pancreas which allows glucose to be transported to the cells to be used as a source of energy for the human body. It is the hormone that allows the accumulation of fat in the body when there is an excess of glucose that is not used by the cells. Diabetics have problems related to this hormone and in some cases must inject it if their pancreas has already suffered damage and does not produce enough of it.

iron: is an important mineral that the body needs to produce hemoglobin, a substance in the blood that carries oxygen from the lungs to tissues throughout the body. Iron is also an important part of many other proteins and enzymes that the body needs for growth and development. Blood is red because of its iron mineral content.

lactic acid: when blood glucose, which is a type of sugar, is fermented it is converted to lactic acid. Lactic acid, like all acids, is a substance that can create corrosion and damage to body tissues. For example, a person does physical exercise and then the muscles ache for several days. This happens due to the accumulation of lactic acid that is generated inside the body during exercise. It is called "lactic" because it was first discovered in milk products and that is why it comes from the word "lactic" (from milk).

metabolic syndrome: when you suffer from INSULIN RESISTANCE, abdominal obesity, high triglycerides and hypertension (high blood pressure) at the same time.

minerals: minerals are very important elements for health since, among other things, they help in the creation of different hormones. Minerals are found in vegetables, salads and soil. Some minerals are magnesium, potassium, and iron.

mitochondria: the mitochondria is the part of a cell that functions like a small furnace that produces energy. When you ingest food, the body breaks it down into very small particles that are transported to the cells. Then the mitochondria picks up those nutrients and mixes them with oxygen, generating combustion, which produces heat energy. That is why, when our metabolism is working well, we feel our body warm. That heat energy is called adenosine triphosphate, or ATP for short. ATP is the body's internal chemical energy, which enables the movement we call life.

Mitochondria

Animal Cell

molecules: the word molecule comes from the word *moles* which means mass. A molecule is a group of at least two atoms joined together. The molecules united form things and depending on the type of atoms that make up the molecule, it will be the type of element that we have. For example, fats are made up of molecules made up of carbon, hydrogen, and oxygen

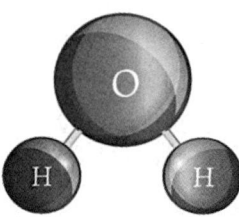
Water Molecule H_2O

organ: an organ is a grouping of cells that form tissues that work together in coordination to perform vital functions in our bodies. Examples of some organs are the stomach, liver, lungs, and heart.

osteoporosis: loss of bone proteins and minerals. As a result, the bone is less resistant and more fragile than normal and breaks relatively easily.

pancreas: is a gland about the size of your fist that is located right next to the stomach, toward the top of the abdomen. The pancreas produces hormones such as insulin and different enzymes to digest carbohydrates, proteins, and fats.

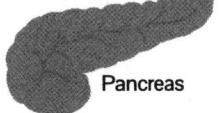

PARASYMPATHETIC Nervous System: that part of the nervous system that slows the heart rate and relaxes the musculature to allow rest and relaxation, or deep, restorative sleep. We also call it Passive Nervous System.

phosphoric acid: a type of acid contained in all soft drinks (including diet soft drinks) such as Coca-Cola and others, which destroys oxygen in the body and reduces metabolism. The phosphoric acid in soft drinks is what causes the "little pins on the tongue feeling" that carbonated soft drinks cause.

physiology: physiology, from the Greek *physis* "nature" and *logos* " knowledge or study". It is the biological science that studies the functioning of living beings.

phytic acid: is a substance that blocks the absorption of essential minerals such as calcium, magnesium, copper, iron and especially the mineral zinc. The mineral zinc has a lot to do with protecting the immune system, improving sexual function in men and preventing prostate cancer.

polyps: a polyp is a small protrusion that can grow in different areas of our body such as the stomach, gallbladder, uterus, vagina, and intestines, among other areas. Most of these growths are benign, but in some cases, if they grow too large, they can cause intestinal obstruction.

polyunsaturated oils: oils and fats are made up of molecules composed of carbon, hydrogen, and oxygen atoms. Polyunsaturated oils contain a large amount of carbon atoms that are not bonded to hydrogen atoms and therefore react to oxygen and can oxidize or rot. These are oils like corn oil, vegetable oil, sunflower oil, etc.

proteins: proteins are foods that provide maximum energy to the body such as meats, seafoods, eggs, cheeses, and proteins such as whey protein. Proteins are composed of amino acids† and have the property that they do not provoke the human body to produce a large amount of insulin as refined carbohydrates (bread, flour, pasta, sugar, etc.)

purines: natural substances contained in DNA (deoxyribonucleic acid), which is the primary storage of hereditary genetic information in all living beings. When purines are used inside the cells, uric acid is produced. Excess uric acid, especially in those with an Excited Nervous System, can produce the inflammatory arthritic type of condition called gout. Foods that are high in purines have an exciting and stimulating effect on the nervous system, as well as causing constriction (narrowing that partially closes capillaries), which can raise blood pressure. Some foods with a high purine content are anchovies, crustaceans, sardines, meat, spinach and mushrooms.

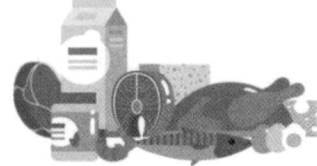

reflux - acidity: when the stomach is irritated, and its acids begin to move up the esophagus (tube leading from the throat to the stomach). This causes burning, irritation, and inflammation of the esophagus.

regimen: a system or method of measuring and controlling the amount and type of food used in the diet.

science: the word science comes from the Latin *scientia* which means "knowledge". Science is an ordered system of structured knowledge that studies, investigates, and interprets natural, social, and artificial phenomena. Scientific knowledge is obtained through observations and experimentation.

sedentary life: also known as sedentarism, is the most common lifestyle. It includes little exercise and tends to increase the incidence of health problems, especially obesity and cardiovascular disease. It is a common lifestyle in modern, highly technological cities, where everything is designed to avoid great physical effort.

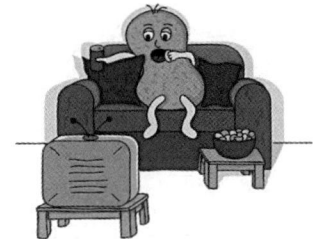

serotonin: a substance produced by the brain that has an antidepressant effect and is considered responsible for causing a good mood.

spinal medulla: this is that large bundle of different nerves that travel from the brain through the entire length of the spinal cord and carry the electrical impulses that control all the movements of the body.

starch: starches are molecules composed of simple sugars which are easily converted by the body into glucose. Carbohydrates that are starches such as potato, or sweet potato among others, are composed of starch. Rice is also a starch.

subclinical hypothyroidism: a type of hypothyroidism that many people have that is not detected by thyroid laboratory tests that measure hormones (TSH, T4, T3). This type of subclinical hypothyroidism is very prevalent among people with obesity who suffer from slow metabolism. There are leading physicians who recognize and treat it. There are other doctors who do not give it any credit and prefer to medicate their patient with an antidepressant that creates more obesity and uncontrolled diabetes anyway.

sweetener: a sweetener is any substance, natural or artificial, that provides a sweet taste to a food or product. Sugar and honey are sweeteners of natural origin, while sucralose or aspartame are sweeteners of artificial origin.

SYMPATHETIC Nervous System: that part of the nervous system that reacts to stress and threats by raising blood pressure, increasing heart rate, and preparing the body to fight or flee. We also call it the Excited Nervous System.

symptoms: a sign, indicator or signal from the body that warns of the existence of a health condition or disease.

synthetic: a synthetic medication is one composed of substances manufactured by the pharmaceutical industry that are not natural to the body.

technology: is the name given to a collection of knowledge that is applied in an orderly manner to achieve desired results or effects. A real technology can always produce predictable results.

thyroid: the thyroid gland is in the neck and is shaped like a butterfly with open wings. This gland produces the hormones that control the metabolism and the body temperature. When this gland fails in its production of hormones, it causes serious disruptions in the health and energy of the body.

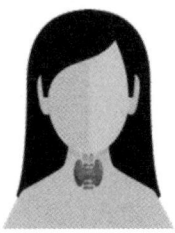

trans-fatty acids: trans-fatty acids are fat molecules that have been damaged and deformed by the process of changing polyunsaturated oils (corn, soy, sunflower, vegetable) from a liquid to a solid state. This process of converting oil into solid fat is called hydrogenation and is carried out by heating the oil to high temperatures while applying electric current and pumping hydrogen gas into it. Because of this, the molecules of trans-fatty oils have lost their normal molecular shape and have become deformed so that the body treats them as if they were toxics. Products such as margarine are full of trans-fatty acids.

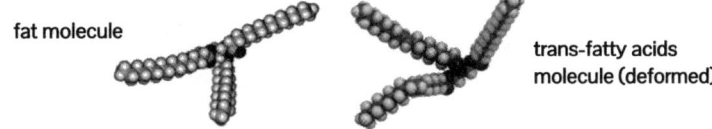

triglycerides: triglycerides are fats that are produced in the liver. When someone is told by their doctor "you have high triglycerides" it means that the person has a lot of fat floating around in their blood, which is extremely dangerous for their health.

tubers: tubers are edible roots, such as potato, sweet potato, and cassava, among many others, which are carbohydrates and increase glucose.

uric acid: is an acid produced by the liver, muscles, intestines, and kidneys when processing purines. If the liver has lost its ability to detoxify the body and eliminate uric acid then diseases such as gout occur, due to over-accumulation of uric acid in the body.

vital: vital means that it is inherent to life or that it is related to it. Vital means that it is indispensable for something to function.

vitamins: vitamins are essential components for life and ingesting them in a balanced way and in essential doses promotes the correct functioning of the body. Most essential vitamins cannot be produced by the body, so the only way to obtain them is through the intake of foods that contain them. Vitamins are nutrients that together with other nutritional elements make all body processes take place.

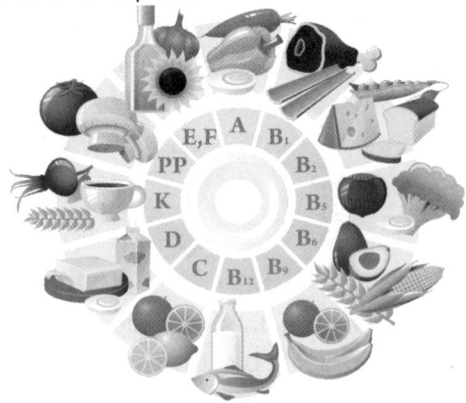

NATURALSLIM® LOCATIONS

To receive professional and personalized help from a Certified Metabolism Consultant, you can contact any of our NaturalSlim centers. We specialize in cases of people who have already experienced several failures, due to slow metabolism, diabetes or hypothyroidism. If you are far away from a NaturalSlim center, call us as we can also offer you remote service and assistance.

NaturalSlim® Puerto Rico
Tel: 787-763-2527
www.NaturalSlimStore.com
On-site consulting in San Juan, Mayaguez, Humacao and Remote Service to all Puerto Rico and the Dominican Republic.

NaturalSlim® United States
Toll Free: 1-888-348-7352
www.us.NaturalSlim.com
On-site consulting in Largo and Orlando, Florida, and Remote Service to all United States and Canada.

NaturalSlim® Panama
Tel: +507 396-6000
www.NaturalSlim.com
On-site consulting and Remote Service to all Panama.

NaturalSlim® Costa Rica
Tel: +506 2430-2010
www.NaturalSlim.com
On-site consulting in Alajuela and Remote Service to all Costa Rica.

NaturalSlim® Colombia
Tel: 57-70-20-928
www.NaturalSlim.com
Remote Service to all Colombia.

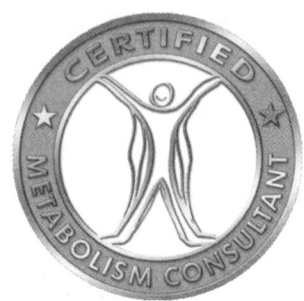

NaturalSlim® Europe
www.Naturalslim.eu
Remote Service in Spain - tel: 646-04-74-32
Remote Service to all Europe – tel: +31-20-2296300

El Poder del Metabolismo Center Curaçao
Tel: +599 9 569 2832
Dr. Isbely Cooper – Salú i Bienestar

ADDITIONAL HELP SITES

MetabolismoTV.com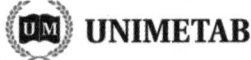
Internet TV channel and interactive video blog about metabolism and health. Watch the latest video episodes where Frank Suárez explains the most interesting topics about his latest discoveries and metabolism technology. You can also watch them on our YouTube.com/MetabolismoTV channel. You can become a member of MetabolismoTV for free, where every week we publish four new videos based on metabolism and health topics. More than 100,000 people visit us every week, looking for information to help them improve their metabolism and health, which, of course, includes getting diabetes under control and avoiding the complications that poorly controlled diabetes can cause. For additional or contact information you can write us at info@metabolismotv.com or you can contact us through MetabolismoTV on Facebook.

Unimetab.com — UNIMETAB
Unimetab is the most complete virtual study center that exists about metabolism and health. Unimetab means "unique metabolism" as with the power of our metabolism we can improve most health conditions, in addition to slimming down. Courses are offered from basic to advanced, based on the research and findings of obesity and metabolism specialist Frank Suárez. The courses have special educational videos made by Frank, exam tests after each lesson, illustrative graphs and photos of each concept, practice exercises, and an official certificate signed by Frank.

The courses can be done on mobile phone, tablet, or computer, at the time that is most convenient for each person 24/7. Course material can be reviewed or used for future reference, as it will continue to be accessible to Unimetab students on permanent basis. Visit us at www.unimetab.com

PreguntaleAFrank.com

Search page for answers to all the questions you may have about metabolism and health. On this website you will find more than a thousand articles in which Frank answers all your questions about health and metabolism topics, with reference to his videos on MetabolismoTV.

DiabetesTV

The revolution in the subject of diabetes. On the DiabetesTV channel on YouTube you will find videos explaining how to control diabetes in a simple and practical way, based on the recommendations of Frank Suárez in his book *Problem-Free Diabetes*. In DiabetesTV, Sylvia Colón, licensed Nutritionist, Dietitian, Diabetes Specialist and Certified Metabolism Consultant, will give you the tools so that diabetes does not control your life and you can slim down and improve your health even if you suffer from this condition.

ADDITIONAL HELP BOOKS

The Power of Your Metabolism

Published in 2006, this book won the International Latino Literary Award as the best health book of 2010. It also received the special "Triple Crown Award" for winning the unanimous vote of the judges. In this book, Frank exposes all the basic facts for the improvement of metabolism and health. *The Power of Your Metabolism* has sold over one million copies worldwide and has been translated into English, French, Dutch and German, with thousands of success stories of people who have achieved their goals by applying the knowledge presented in this book.

In a world of controversy about obesity, *The Power of Your Metabolism* records the techniques and factors that help restore metabolism, based on the experience and observations of what has worked for hundreds of thousands of people. The techniques for losing weight naturally are described in this Best-Seller. Topics include a diet you can live with, why fats are not to blame for obesity, the difference between losing weight and slimming down, foods that are sources of energy for the metabolism, and the candida albicans yeast, among others. The book defines the causes and solutions to the problem of slow metabolism that has some people "dieting for life" while others are skinny no matter what they eat. Therefore, it concludes that losing weight is not only about what you eat.

You can purchase this book at:
NaturalSlim Centers
Amazon (Digital & Printed Version)
MetabolismoTVBooks.com

Problem-Free Diabetes

The book *Problem-Free Diabetes, Controlling Diabetes with the Help of The Power of Your Metabolism*, is the result of Frank Suárez 's research work of more than 5 years. It is a book written for diabetic patients, for family caregivers and for physicians or health professionals who want to see their patients improve without the need to continue increasing doses of medications or the risks of health complications. It contains 561 pages of explanations, in simple language, on all the aspects that need to be understood to achieve diabetes control. As diabetes is a disease that can be fatal, this book has the main purpose of avoiding the health problems and complications (loss of eyesight, kidney damage, etc.) that can result from poorly controlled diabetes.

The book contains 175 photos, diagrams, and illustrations to help in the understanding of the subject. Due to the seriousness of the subject, in *Problem-Free Diabetes*, Frank Suárez references a total of 965 clinical studies, books, scientific articles and doctors' opinions that endorse the explanations he offers to the reader. In addition, the book includes a glossary (definitions of words) that explains in a simple way the 124 most important words or medical terms that need to be understood in the subject of diabetes. The goal of the book is to have a patient or family member of a diabetic patient educated and responsibly contributing to the management of diabetes by assisting their physician or other qualified health care professional in monitoring their condition. *Problem-Free Diabetes* is an education tool that will contribute to the control of diabetes and to the reduction of medical costs wherever it is applied.

You can purchase this book at:
NaturalSlim Centers
Amazon (Digital & Printed Version)
MetabolismoTVBooks.com

The Way to Happiness Booklet

The booklet *The Way to Happiness* is a non-religious moral code based entirely on common sense. It was written by L. Ron Hubbard as an individual work and is not part of any religious doctrine. Frank Suárez, *The Power of Your Metabolism*, MetabolismoTV and NaturalSlim proudly support and recommend knowing the moral values promoted and taught by *The Way to Happiness Foundation* (thewaytohappiness.org).

We cannot separate health from moral values, since the first precept of *The Way to Happiness* is to **Take Care of Yourself**. It is a moral obligation of every person, every parent, grandparent, or loved one to know the principles that preserve and care for health.

The lack of this basic health knowledge, as taught in the book *The Power of Your Metabolism*, has caused the public to suffer from excessive overweight, obesity, diabetes, high blood pressure, poor sleep quality, lack of energy and mental problems.

After more than twenty years of helping hundreds of thousands of people, it is Frank Suárez 's opinion that ignorance about the basics of metabolism and health keeps the world's population sick, full of symptoms and with multiple conditions of bad health that require excessive medications, simply because there is no genuine interest in caring for the public to maintain the sales and income of the pharmaceutical empire and the medical industry.

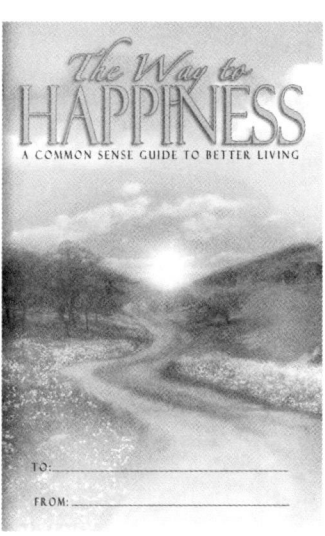

This has happened because of a lack of morals in those who direct medical education and in those who plan to further medicate our children, loved ones and the elderly every day. That is why it is important to share moral values that are based on common sense and that promote that we can live happier.

You can obtain free copies of this booklet at:
NaturalSlim Centers
or TheWayToHappiness.org

ADVISORS AND SPECIALISTS

Dr. Carlos M. Cidre Miranda
Internist, American Board of Internal Medicine Diplomate, Principal Consultant Physician for NaturalSlim

Urb. Atenas Elliot Vélez B-41
Manatí, Puerto Rico
Tel: 787-884-3139

Bayamón Medical Plaza Ste. 303
Bayamón, Puerto Rico
Tel: 787-780-6680
787-786-4627

Dr. Carlos Cidre is the consulting physician for the NaturalSlim System. He is an internist, Board Certified, with over 30 years of experience and who has had extensive experience treating hundreds of diabetic patients many of whom with his help were able to reduce or eliminate the use of medications including injected insulin. Dr. Cidre's goal has been to educate his diabetic patients to empower them and in doing so make them active participants in the management of their diabetic condition. Dr. Cidre has been certified as a Certified Metabolic Consultant (CMC) by the NaturalSlim System for several years reason why he perfectly knows the metabolic restoration technology expressed in this book.

Dr. Ramón Crespo Almeida
Internist and Specialist in Health Administration
Consultant Physician for NaturalSlim Mexico

Dr. Crespo has spent his entire life dedicated to helping people with their health and managing health systems, both in his native Cuba as well as in Mexico. Currently, he helps his patients improve their health conditions by applying the metabolism restoration techniques, with great success in his practice. Dr. Crespo is the consulting physician for NaturalSlim in Mexico City.

Sylvia M. Colón
Licensed Nutritionist, Dietitian L.N.D.
Diabetes Educator
Nutriwise Team • email: scnutriwise@gmail.com

Nutritionist/Dietitian consultant of the NaturalSlim System and the book *Problem-Free Diabetes*. Licensed Nutritionist Colón is a Certified Metabolism Consultant. She assists in Community Education programs and training programs for other health professionals. Sylvia educates on the use of metabolic restoration technology for conditions related to obesity and diabetes. In addition, she publishes educational videos about diabetes, based on the book *Problem-Free Diabetes*, on the YouTube channel DiabetesTV.

Viridiana Martínez
Licensed Nutritionist, Certified Metabolism Consultant and Director of the Diabetes Management Program from the Red Cross of Coahuila, México

Doctor in Nutrition Viridiana Martinez has led efforts to control the incidence of diabetes in the state of Coahuila, Mexico. Since 2013 she has successfully directed the Diabetes Control Program at the Red Cross in this state. With her dedicated work, she has helped hundreds of people manage their diabetes problem using the 3x1 Diet and metabolism restoration technology.

Thematic Index

2x1 Diet .... V, 10
3x1 Diet . III, V, VII, 10, XVI, 56, 112, 113, 119, 125, 126, 128, 129, 131, 132, 133, 135, 139, 140, 142, 144, 145, 154, 159, 160, 164, 197, 202, 233, 239, 242, 253, 264, 272, 274, 288, 300, 302, 325, 357
acetaminophen 49, 50, 325
acidity .. 34, 54, 102, 285, 286, 287, 289, 305, 326, 343
addiction .. 34, 131, 159, 160, 161, 163, 262, 265
adrenals 37, 100, 106, 225, 299, 326, 332
Aggressor Foods XVI, 173, 201, 202, 205, 206, 207, 209, 210
alcoholic beverages 91, 121
allergies 156, 180, 181, 183, 279, 327
amino acids 64, 198, 305, 327, 342
anabolics 321
antibiotic 273, 276
antidepressant . 48, 50, 135, 160, 183, 191, 223, 296, 317, 318, 343, 344
anxiety IV, 45, 57, 151, 159, 208, 210, 291, 296, 313, 320
arrhythmia 53, 101, 296, 331
arteries 42, 66, 68, 323, 327, 328
arthritis 42, 53, 149, 151, 153, 211, 258, 299, 300, 302, 328, 336
aspartame 42, 45, 46, 50, 344
asthmatics 300
atherosclerosis 66, 328
atoms 33, 39, 83, 84, 188, 192, 328, 340, 342
ATP 85, 86, 328, 340
attention deficit 151, 156
autoimmune .. 53, 222, 299, 311, 313, 329
Autonomous Nervous System ... 97, 100, 102, 103, 104, 112, 115, 138, 329
avocado oil 39
biological individuality . 56, 137, 325, 329
blood pressure ... III, IV, VI, 29, 48, 49, 54, 61, 66, 67, 72, 82, 91, 92, 93, 97, 102, 106, 140, 142, 149, 151, 153, 208, 247, 292, 294, 295, 296, 306, 323, 324, 328, 329, 333, 337, 339, 342, 344, 353
body temperature ... 29, 35, 100, 101, 188, 192, 193, 194, 198, 338, 345
brain 48, 53, 66, 97, 98, 99, 100, 102, 106, 115, 150, 151, 155, 159, 160, 183, 188, 196, 197, 261, 312, 328, 329, 333, 343
bread 31, 32, 35, 55, 64, 120, 131, 139, 141, 143, 156, 159, 161, 181, 189, 190, 204, 208, 331, 342
breakfast. 55, 57, 124, 133, 145, 165, 264, 265, 303, 305, 306, 316
butter 40, 41, 120, 121, 122, 206, 209, 227
calcium .. 47, 66, 105, 295, 309, 328, 341
calm the nervous system 153, 154, 173, 313
calories 43, 55, 56, 62, 63, 64, 69, 72, 80, 119, 275, 330
cancer ..... VI, XV, XVI, 27, 47, 49, 149, 151, 153, 178, 180, 190, 206, 208, 210, 211, 216, 217, 222, 258, 282, 283, 307, 311, 312, 330, 341
candida albicans ... 156, 163, 177, 178, 179, 182, 184, 250, 265, 271, 274, 276, 277, 278, 316, 330, 351
candida yeast XVI, 154, 156, 163, 177, 178, 179, 180, 181, 182, 183, 184, 185, 242, 250, 251, 254, 265, 271, 272, 273, 274, 276, 277, 278, 301, 316, 330, 335, 351
candidiasis 156, 177, 183, 210, 222
Candiseptic Kit 271, 273, 274
canola oil 39
carbonated soft drinks ... 45, 46, 121, 156, 159, 341
cardiac palpitations 101, 331
cascara sagrada. 280
Central Nervous System . 56, 98, 99, 311, 315, 325
cheese 31, 122, 161, 209
cheeses 64, 113, 122, 132, 139, 161, 162, 164, 206, 227, 327, 342

359

children... 42, 43, 52, 155, 156, 206, 235, 244, 314, 320, 335, 353
cholesterol....III, V, 29, 40, 41, 52, 53, 66, 72, 82, 188, 191, 192, 226, 247, 331, 334
circadian.. 170, 331
clinical studies... 43, 200, 227, 276, 284, 301, 306, 323, 332, 352
Coco-10 Plus 275, 276, 277, 278, 304, 306
cold extremities 35, 48, 180, 188, 191, 338
colorants 38, 41, 156
combustible 29, 32, 107, 136, 138, 147, 241, 285, 332, 335, 336
constipation 28, 35, 92, 93, 101, 107, 108, 110, 113, 149, 151, 180, 188, 191, 210, 279, 280, 295, 296, 338
Constipend.................................... 279, 280
CoQ10 275
corn..... 31, 32, 33, 39, 40, 42, 43, 44, 50, 55, 90, 120, 121, 131, 139, 205, 206, 209, 214, 331, 335, 342, 345
corn syrup.............. 42, 43, 44, 50, 90, 121
cortisol XXII, 37, 38, 69, 137, 162, 170, 171, 172, 175, 220, 228, 299, 300, 302, 319, 320, 324, 326, 332
cortisone 300, 332
cystitis 180
depression IV, 35, 45, 47, 48, 49, 53, 151, 153, 180, 183, 188, 190, 191, 194, 206, 210, 291, 338
desayuno 195, 196
detox 132, 159, 162, 163, 164, 265
diabetes...... III, IV, VI, XVI, XXIII, 28, 29, 31, 41, 43, 47, 48, 52, 53, 55, 56, 61, 70, 79, 81, 82, 86, 87, 92, 93, 95, 105, 110, 112, 113, 119, 125, 126, 131, 132, 148, 149, 151, 153, 159, 168, 173, 191, 199, 200, 201, 202, 203, 204, 206, 210, 211, 214, 217, 242, 275, 276, 288, 289, 294, 295, 302, 303, 305, 307, 308, 310, 318, 319, 320, 321, 324, 325, 330, 333, 344, 347, 349, 350, 352, 353, 356, 357
diabetic... III, VI, 97, 114, 119, 131, 200, 201, 202, 203, 204, 205, 210, 211, 212, 271, 274, 285, 300, 324, 329, 333, 352, 355
diabetic neuropathy ... XVI, 53, 299, 302, 333

diabetics 33, 35, 43, 113, 131, 135, 200, 203, 204, 205, 291, 306, 316, 318, 339
diarrhea 101, 163, 180, 250, 251, 273, 277, 278, 297, 298, 299
digestion. 28, 48, 49, 88, 91, 93, 97, 100, 102, 108, 110, 140, 151, 284, 285, 286, 287, 288, 289, 305, 329, 333
digestive problems... 111, 116, 149, 188, 191, 210, 285, 286, 289, 305, 338
diuretic 67, 91, 333
edema 222
eggs.... 64, 66, 72, 132, 139, 161, 162, 164, 209, 225, 327, 342
enzymes......... 47, 65, 188, 287, 288, 289, 305, 309, 334, 339, 341
estrogen 29, 188, 219, 220, 221, 222, 223, 228, 281, 282, 283, 321, 331, 334
Excited Nervous System ... 103, 105, 106, 107, 108, 109, 110, 111, 113, 115, 116, 138, 139, 140, 141, 142, 143, 147, 148, 149, 150, 151, 152, 153, 155, 156, 157, 158, 161, 167, 173, 174, 205, 295, 297, 311, 312, 314, 315, 342, 344
exercise .... III, 10, 28, 34, 53, 80, 179, 216, 231, 232, 233, 234, 235, 236, 237, 238, 239, 249, 258, 261, 267, 339, 343
fatigue....... 45, 48, 52, 180, 183, 193, 291, 296
Femme Balance......... 281, 282, 283, 284
fiber... 32, 334
fibroids 222
fibromyalgia 222
fish 63, 64, 66, 113, 122, 132, 139, 143, 148, 161, 327
fluoride...................... 47, 48, 50, 190, 336
fruit juices 42, 43, 44, 88, 90, 131
fruits 32, 44, 121, 122, 131, 139, 141, 292
gases.... 53, 180, 181, 285, 286, 289, 305
genetically modified 43, 214, 335
glasses of water 87, 88, 93, 157, 263
glucagon 123, 124, 125, 137, 163, 336
glucose ... III, VI, VII, 29, 31, 32, 33, 34, 35, 37, 42, 53, 57, 64, 65, 66, 79, 91, 97, 106, 107, 113, 114, 119, 120, 121, 123, 124, 125, 126, 131, 132, 135, 172, 175, 183, 203, 204, 205, 206, 207, 209, 210, 211, 212, 213, 214, 217, 241, 243, 244, 245, 246, 249, 251, 253, 261,

296, 329, 331, 333, 334, 336, 338, 339, 344, 346
glycogen 107, 336
goitrogens 47, 48, 189, 336
hamburgers 31, 58, 77
heart...29, 36, 41, 42, 45, 48, 54, 66, 68, 97, 99, 100, 101, 102, 103, 106, 115, 151, 206, 208, 225, 227, 296, 327, 328, 329, 331, 337, 340, 341, 344
Helpzymes 284, 286, 287, 288
homeostasis 96, 337
hormone XXII, 29, 34, 37, 38, 47, 48, 64, 65, 67, 69, 105, 123, 124, 162, 163, 170, 171, 172, 175, 188, 219, 220, 221, 222, 223, 224, 225, 226, 234, 235, 241, 244, 245, 281, 282, 299, 300, 302, 317, 319, 322, 323, 324, 326, 331, 332, 334, 336, 337, 339
hormones 29, 34, 35, 37, 47, 48, 65, 137, 151, 170, 187, 188, 189, 191, 192, 196, 197, 198, 219, 221, 226, 228, 244, 317, 319, 321, 326, 331, 337, 338, 340, 341, 344, 345
Hyperactivity 155
hypertension .XVI, 29, 49, 52, 61, 68, 72, 151, 201, 291, 292, 293, 295, 337, 339
hyperthyroidism 48, 113, 190, 337
hypoglycemia 53, 306, 338
hypothyroidism.... XVI, 29, 31, 35, 48, 52, 53, 113, 141, 187, 191, 192, 193, 194, 195, 198, 206, 210, 266, 286, 297, 308, 318, 338, 344, 347
immune system ...VI, 28, 47, 53, 101, 108, 156, 178, 182, 225, 309, 327, 329, 341
insomniaXVI, 35, 45, 48, 52, 53, 110, 135, 140, 149, 151, 191, 206, 296, 297, 313, 319, 320, 337
insulin .III, 34, 35, 42, 49, 53, 56, 64, 65, 123, 124, 125, 131, 137, 163, 201, 202, 204, 214, 224, 241, 242, 243, 244, 245, 246, 247, 253, 255, 288, 294, 295, 305, 325, 336, 338, 339, 341, 342, 355
Intermittent Fasting 247, 248, 249, 250, 251, 252, 253, 254, 255, 256, 267
intestinal flora 177, 182, 272, 273
iodine 188, 189, 190, 192, 196, 317
itchy skin 163, 180, 251, 272, 277
Kadsorb........................290, 291, 292, 293

lactic acid.. 34, 339
libido.............................. XVI, 222, 223, 283
liver29, 37, 41, 42, 49, 51, 54, 61, 97, 100, 106, 107, 108, 115, 122, 124, 182, 224, 249, 261, 329, 336, 340, 345, 346
lupus 222
lymphatic system 51
MagicMag 162, 280, 294, 297, 298, 320
maltitol 122
margarine 40, 41, 50, 345
meat....... 31, 105, 111, 113, 122, 138, 140, 141, 142, 144, 148, 221, 227, 342
medications ... III, IV, V, VI, 10, XVI, 29, 48, 49, 50, 62, 80, 82, 135, 156, 182, 183, 199, 200, 201, 202, 203, 208, 216, 227, 238, 271, 282, 284, 286, 287, 291, 295, 296, 300, 301, 302, 325, 338, 352, 353, 355
menopause...282
menstruation.......180, 210, 220, 222, 223
MetabOil 299, 301, 302
metabolic balance .96, 101, 102, 108, 132, 137
Metabolic Protein..... 303, 304, 305, 306
metabolic syndrome 49, 339
Metabolic Vitamins..................................310
milk....31, 34, 48, 55, 88, 90, 121, 122, 131, 161, 204, 206, 281, 303, 339
minerals 47, 54, 68, 69, 105, 196, 198, 249, 259, 261, 284, 303, 307, 308, 309, 310, 316, 317, 339, 341
mitochondria 85, 187, 328, 340
multiple sclerosis 222, 302
muscle spasms........................... 291, 296
muscles34, 42, 69, 70, 97, 100, 106, 107, 115, 123, 219, 225, 226, 231, 234, 235, 336, 337, 339, 346
musculature 103, 220, 227, 234, 235, 341
nervous system ..XVI, 36, 48, 49, 79, 80, 97, 98, 99, 102, 103, 105, 106, 108, 109, 110, 111, 112, 113, 114, 115, 116, 117, 132, 135, 137, 138, 140, 141, 142, 143, 144, 145, 147, 149, 151, 153, 154, 156, 157, 159, 161, 162, 164, 165, 167, 169, 173, 174, 183, 196, 206, 210, 212, 227, 239, 261, 264, 265, 281, 291, 295, 313, 318, 320, 325, 329, 341, 342, 344
niacin 317
niacinamide 317

olive oil 39, 122, 139
osteoporosis 54, 222, 296, 341
oxygen 32, 33, 34, 39, 46, 47, 51, 83, 84, 85, 92, 100, 187, 188, 193, 194, 197, 285, 328, 332, 335, 339, 340, 341, 342
pancreas 34, 56, 65, 97, 100, 108, 115, 123, 124, 325, 329, 336, 339, 341
Parasympathetic Nervous System... 103, 341
Passive Nervous System... 103, 105, 108, 109, 110, 111, 113, 138, 139, 141, 142, 143, 144, 147, 148, 149, 150, 151, 167, 169, 175, 295, 311, 312, 313, 314, 341
Peripheral Nervous System .. 98, 99, 100
phosphoric acid 46, 341
physiology 104, 341
polyunsaturated oils 39, 40, 50, 342, 345
pork 63, 64, 111, 122, 132, 139, 140, 141, 142, 161, 206, 209, 327
potassium 47, 105, 154, 157, 189, 249, 250, 290, 291, 292, 293, 294, 296, 340
preservatives 38, 156
progesterone 220, 221, 222, 223, 281, 282, 283, 284, 321
proteins 47, 54, 64, 65, 139, 161, 188, 259, 284, 286, 287, 288, 289, 305, 327, 334, 339, 341, 342
refined carbohydrates XVI, 31, 32, 33, 34, 35, 49, 54, 57, 58, 61, 64, 65, 68, 72, 77, 90, 119, 123, 141, 143, 144, 159, 160, 161, 162, 163, 164, 177, 178, 182, 183, 184, 189, 190, 193, 197, 224, 255, 262, 265, 274, 275, 277, 300, 301, 306, 310, 320, 330, 331, 335, 342
reflux .... XVI, 54, 285, 287, 338, 343
RelaxSlim 10, 315, 316, 317, 318, 319
rice V, 31, 32, 33, 42, 53, 55, 63, 65, 77, 120, 131, 141, 161, 181, 204, 206, 207, 209, 213, 217, 331, 338, 344
serotonin 160, 343
sex 180, 191, 223, 225, 228, 323
sexual ..... XVI, 47, 48, 53, 89, 92, 93, 103, 151, 202, 222, 225, 227, 283, 318, 323, 324, 333, 334, 341
sinus 49, 180, 181, 183, 325
soy 33, 39, 40, 47, 48, 50, 120, 122, 141, 189, 209, 336, 345

spinal medulla 98, 343
starches. 42, 123, 159, 183, 190, 275, 277, 344
stevia 46, 90, 122
stress XVI, 36, 37, 38, 50, 52, 57, 58, 59, 69, 77, 102, 137, 149, 150, 151, 160, 162, 168, 170, 172, 196, 197, 205, 206, 210, 212, 214, 217, 220, 227, 228, 262, 295, 296, 299, 300, 302, 316, 318, 319, 320, 321, 324, 326, 332, 344
Stress Defender 319, 320
sucralose 42, 46, 344
sugar IV, VI, 29, 31, 32, 33, 34, 41, 42, 43, 45, 51, 53, 64, 90, 91, 119, 121, 122, 126, 131, 132, 139, 141, 155, 156, 161, 172, 203, 209, 212, 241, 277, 291, 305, 310, 331, 333, 336, 338, 339, 342, 344
sweetener 42, 45, 50, 344
sweets .31, 32, 96, 131, 139, 143, 155, 159, 181, 305, 306, 320, 331
Sympathetic Nervous System .. 102, 103, 344
T3 hormone 188, 317
T4 hormone 188, 189, 317
TAM 209
tequila 91
Testosterin 227, 321, 323
testosterone 29, 34, 219, 220, 223, 224, 225, 226, 227, 228, 282, 322, 323, 324, 331, 337
thyroid VII, XV, 28, 29, 35, 39, 47, 48, 49, 56, 63, 100, 106, 113, 141, 149, 151, 154, 187, 188, 189, 190, 191, 192, 193, 194, 196, 197, 198, 201, 254, 266, 286, 308, 316, 317, 319, 336, 337, 338, 344, 345
toxics 28, 40, 51, 92, 107, 163, 179, 184, 250, 272, 276, 277, 280, 317, 330, 345
trampoline 234, 236, 237, 238
trans-fatty acids 40, 41, 50, 345
triglycerides III, IV, XVI, 29, 31, 42, 49, 52, 54, 82, 275, 276, 339, 345
TSH hormone 48, 189
tubers 31, 131, 346
Type F Foods ..56, 119, 120, 124, 125, 126, 131, 132, 133, 159, 160, 163, 184, 190, 197, 203, 217, 224, 241, 243, 246, 250, 275, 301, 325

Type S Foods ... 56, 119, 122, 125, 126, 131, 132, 133, 325
uric acid 42, 142, 336, 342, 346
vaginal 54, 90, 163, 177, 180, 182, 183, 222, 272, 274
vaginal discharge 163, 180, 183
vegetable juices .. 132, 154, 157, 247, 290
vegetables 31, 32, 40, 43, 44, 47, 63, 65, 105, 121, 122, 132, 139, 143, 148, 161, 290, 292, 293, 310, 331, 340
vitamins 39, 68, 69, 72, 105, 196, 198, 259, 261, 284, 303, 307, 308, 309, 310, 316, 317, 346
wheat. III, 33, 120, 131, 139, 156, 190, 204, 206, 208, 209, 217
whey 64, 304, 305, 306, 342

NOTES

NOTES